Yes You Can!

Yes You Can!

Rosalie Kaufman
with Daniel Myerson and Didi Fujita

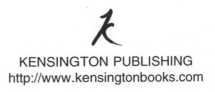

KENSINGTON PUBLISHING
http://www.kensingtonbooks.com

KENSINGTON BOOKS are published by

Kensington Publishing Corp.
850 Third Avenue
New York, NY 10022

Library of Congress Card Catalog Number: 98-066720
ISBN 1-57566-385-6

First Printing: February, 1999
10 9 8 7 6 5 4 3 2 1

Printed in the United States of America

This book is dedicated to Noah Lukeman, our agent, without whose guidance it never would have been written.

Contents

Yes You Can!

CHAPTER ONE

Where I'm Coming From

"Success is the ability to go from failure to failure without loss of enthusiasm."
—Winston Churchill

"Though no one can make a new start, if we begin again, we can make a new finish."
—Anonymous

"There is no failure except no longer trying. Giving up. We all fall, but we don't have to fail."
—Rosalie Kaufman, Group Leader

I don't care if someone is fat. I don't care if someone comes to me and is happy and three hundred pounds overweight. I say to them, fine! Live and be well! But it's when they're miserable, when they can't stand being themselves anymore—that's when I tell them there's another way. People wouldn't go to Weight Watchers® or pick up this book if they were happy. They've usually come to the end of a long, hard road of suffering with their weight.

That was me. For me, springtime meant "the unveiling". I had to take off the heavy coat, I had to display my body in front of all the neighbors who I knew were talking about me. Even if they weren't, I heard them. I had only one goal: it wasn't to write the great American novel, it wasn't to be First Lady—it was to get out of my maternity clothes, and I wasn't even pregnant!

I had worn them all winter because nothing else fit. But winter was coming to an end and I dreaded what the summer would reveal. So on a gloomy day late in February, I finished what I've come to call The Last Supper. It's that meal before the diet begins, the memorial meal. All dieters know what I'm talking about. For some, it's a three-layer box of chocolates, for others it's the wedding cake minus the guests. In my particular case—I'm not ashamed to tell you—it was three weeks of nonstop eating ending with an entire can of whipped cream squirted directly into the mouth, with the firm belief that this was the last time I would ever taste whipped cream. This phenomenon of The Last Supper is based on a common error. Dieters get into an I'll-never-eat-sugar-again state of mind. They become grim. Fanatical. "This is my last piece of cake."

When I hear those words, I know that person is doomed. Doomed. Why? Because the body and the mind are going to rebel. What goes up must come down. You can live on water and celery for just so long and then you're back where you started. To succeed over a long period of time, you must have something to sustain you, a long-term game plan. Extreme resolutions don't last, whether they relate to food, exercise, or any other aspect of your weight plan. For example, in one of my groups a very heavy woman who hadn't exercised for years decided after a two-day binge that this was *it!* She was so motivated by a meeting on exercise that she decided to walk home—a good distance of about thirty blocks. Halfway there, she had to slump over a mailbox for support and a police car stopped to make sure she was okay. When she finally got home, hours later, exhausted and in pain, she was demoralized. As far as I know, that was the end of her exercise program at that particular time. In my own way, my Last Supper resolutions were just as extreme.

So, desperate to do something for myself, I grabbed my protesting three-year-old and marched up the stairs to a Weight Watchers® meeting. Just my bad luck. The receptionist that day was a slim, lovely redhead. I wanted to turn around and walk right out. She's no former Weight Watchers® member, I thought. It's all a lie. What kept me there? Someone even heavier than I was coming up behind me, huffing and puffing as if she had just run the four-minute mile. Two things went through my mind: *That's me in two years, if I keep going on this way,* and the inspirational thought: *If she can do it, so can I.*

The next step, after signing in and paying dues, was the weigh-in. I should have left my son at home with a baby-sitter and made this my hour for myself. It would have been especially good to be alone for the first shock, the bad news. I'd put off and put off that moment of truth. I hadn't wanted to know. Like so many others, my idea was, *First lose weight, then go on the scale.* Having the right attitude about the scale can make you or break you—but that's for later.

The ladies and men (there were men, even though it was day-time—and I give them special credit) were taking off everything they could take off: earrings, complicated girdle systems, jewelry, belts, shoes—one zealot even took off her wig. And even without— well, let's say without *something*—I still weighed more than I had imagined possible. I knew it was bad, because none of my clothes fit, but the exact dimensions of the disaster had escaped me. I was ten pounds heavier than my "peak" weight.

So what would a typical person's reaction be? To start dieting? If that's your answer, you don't know the first thing about dieting and losing weight. The first response is: *All is lost. I'll never get it off. Let me go home and eat something and then I'll think about losing weight.*

Then starts the litany of recriminations: *How did I let it get so out of hand? Why didn't I stop sooner?* And there is good reason for desperation: facing the need to lose a lot of weight is like facing Mount Everest and wondering how to begin the climb. We have a long road ahead of us, but we all want to be thin yesterday. We imagine the horror in our friends' eyes when they see what's become of us; we imagine the class reunion or the family get-together— and since there's no way we can get the weight off in a month, there's no incentive to start.

Again I was on the point of giving up and going on a major binge. But then, thank God, an old saying of my grandmother's came to mind: *If you stink from garlic, does that mean eat more garlic?* She was right!

The next thought that flashed through my mind as I peered through the door and saw the group leader for the first time was, "What does *she* know?" There she stood—in front of thirty peo-ple—stylish suit, perfect hairdo, slender and trim. I listened to her as I had listened to many leaders in the past. I always thought I was smarter than the leader, up on all the latest weight loss techniques. This time a new thought came to me: *How come I'm smart and fat and she's dumb and thin?* So I became a little humble . . .

I realized that the problem was beyond me, and that I would have to make a leap of faith. A friend who loved physics always used to quote Einstein: *You can't get out of a problem using the same thinking you used to get into it.* I had gotten to where I was by following all my impulses and going with my emotions. Maybe it was time to study some of the perspectives of people who hadn't just lost fifty or sixty pounds, but had kept it off for many years— people who had actually changed their lifestyles and life patterns, people who had learned from their mistakes.

Nobody's Saying It's Easy

Nobody's saying it's easy—I've seen some pretty heroic behavior during my twenty-two years as a group leader. Take a mother of four children, working part-time, behind on all the bills, putting aside money to hire a baby-sitter and to take two busses to come to Weight Watchers® on a typical Brooklyn summer's day—hotter than Bangkok. For days she has gone without the massive doses of sugar that are her cure-all. She gets on the scale. Not only hasn't she lost weight, she's gained a quarter of a pound.

Who knows why? There are many possibilities. Water retention, the vegetables she's been eating—I won't go into all the possibilities. Her first thoughts are, *This diet doesn't work—I knew it— I have to go back to starving myself . . .* or *Since I'm gaining weight anyway, at least I should enjoy myself. I'll go out and have that lemon meringue pie.*

Do you realize the strength of will she needs to stop and think and say "no" and go on until something finally gives? Because if she goes back to her old patterns, this woman is entering a vicious cycle. The moment she says "no," she is a hero.

But my first day at Weight Watchers®, I wasn't ready for heroism. And in the beginning, there was no need for it: I lost weight the first week. Not as much as I had hoped, but the number went down. And I was happy. The second week, more. The third week, my weight remained the same. The fifth week, I gained weight after a great week on the program. I wanted to drop out. This had happened so many times in the past. I went to Weight Watchers® two and three times a year for eleven years. I was what people called a *failure*.

I hate that word and I'll tell you why. The word *failure* suggests something that's hopeless, finished. Foolishly, we call it *failure* when we don't live up to our own expectations. And so we become hysterical, we pull out our hair. We think that we are destined to be fat, that we will be fat for the rest of our lives. For some people (fortunately, I wasn't one of them) their entire identity is destroyed in the process. They begin to feel worthless in all areas of their life. Their entire self-image depends on their weight.

What I didn't realize was that those many attempts at Weight Watchers® were preparing the ground. I was learning my own strength and gauging the difficulty of the problem. A man once said to me, "Look at what a failure I am! I ate eight chocolate bars in a night! And that's after months and months of trying." And I said, "What I hear is that *you're counting*. You're counting the number of bars you ate!" Before he started Weight Watchers®, he grabbed food without thinking. He didn't know what he was putting into his mouth. The fact is that after months of keeping a diary of everything he ate, he had become more conscious. That was a big step forward, which he couldn't even see because he was too busy calling himself a failure instead of building on his success.

The point is that these new techniques we learn take a long time to become part of us, and we don't realize that the growth takes place very slowly, over months, sometimes years. We focus on the negative and we give up. If someone came into Weight Watchers® and sat down next to you and said, "I have a really difficult problem"—whatever it is, a tough boss, a sick relative, it doesn't matter what—"and I just couldn't stay on the program this week," would you speak to that person as harshly as you speak to yourself? Would you say to that person, "You're hopeless. You'll never lose weight?" Of course not. Why don't you begin to show yourself a little bit of the charity and understanding you show others?

One of the first steps I took toward health was to become aware of the self-talk that went on after an eating binge. The names I called myself, the body language. I would slump over, hold my arms across my stomach, hide in the back of rooms—I lost all self-respect and dignity. Learning how to overcome this kind of post-binge despair—and binges will occur, because weight loss is not an overnight process—is part of what we'll talk about.

So now I think back to myself again, trudging up those steps in Queens with a three-year-old in one hand and a cheese Danish in the other, barely able to move from a Last Supper that outdid any that preceded it, wearing a maternity dress because nothing else fit. But this time with the realization that it was not enough to change my food plan or go on a diet. I had to change my entire approach. I had to change my life.

I had to take a step back and look at my life seriously. During one of those early Weight Watchers® meetings, our group leader asked, "How did you gain your weight?" I didn't want to discuss my innermost thoughts publicly at the meetings then, but strangely enough, I realized that I had never asked myself that very basic question. Just realizing how it had happened gave me more power over the conditions of my life.

Not that I shared it with anyone. In those days, I could talk during the meeting, but not about my deepest feelings. But I remember the "day" I gained fifty pounds. I was nineteen years old and just married. Eleven months after I got married, I had my first baby. She was the kind of baby who could have driven Dr. Spock crazy. She slept for twenty minutes three times a day, so that she could wake up and start crying again. She was colicky, she was fussy, she was allergic to milk, and I thought probably to me as well. And I was a young girl! Before I got married, I was going to seminary, I was going to school, I was always on the go . . . And all of a sudden, I had to spend the whole day in the house! My in-laws lived in the same building and every afternoon they would come over to give me advice. Well, one day I saw a recipe for lemon meringue pie in *McCall's* magazine.

I'm not dumb! I can follow instructions! The pie came out beautifully. When my husband came home, he said, "Did you save one slice for me?" But I had been in the house all day and he had been out in the world in his clean suit and his hat. No, I didn't have a slice for him. I ate that whole pie myself. And that's how I put on my fifty pounds—that was the beginning of the end.

That was my particular story, but there are as many ways to start overeating as there are people. What sets us off? That is what we have to discover. It could be many things. You have a wedding next week. You've been losing at an average of one pound a week, sometimes staying at the same weight for a whole week. But suddenly you're seized by a desire to look good, very good, at the wedding.

What could be the harm, you ask yourself, if you cut back drastically for a few days so you could lose five pounds before the wedding? So you starve yourself for a day, and at the end of that day, you are so hungry that you lose control and eat nonstop. The result is that instead of losing five pounds, you gain five pounds. You're a victim of your own impatience.

Or take a second example. Your daughter asks you to baby sit for her children during the time you've put aside for a Weight Watchers® meeting, a movie, a walk, whatever. You say, yes. But not having whatever was nourishing to you results in you "giving to yourself" by eating sweets.

RULE: A BANKRUPT PERSON CANNOT GIVE ANY-THING TO ANYONE. LEARN HOW TO SAY "NO."

It's a holiday, and you know that every year around this time you end up bingeing for a week or two. Instead of preparing for the holiday, you stumble into the holiday season, once again without planning, without preparing, without giving it proper thought or attention. How to deal with all the emotions that the holiday brings up and all the situations that spell doom for you?

Or say you've lost your weight and have been doing well on maintenance. But suddenly it occurs to you that you could look better—after all, as the saying goes, you can't be too rich or too thin. Who's ever satisfied? Remember Natalie Wood? She was a petite woman, just about my size. A beautiful woman. Do you know how much she weighed? Ninety-eight pounds! For me, that would be an unrealistic goal—to try to achieve that weight would be self-sabotage and I know it. I've *learned* over the years to keep away from that particular pitfall, but so many others stumble into it after achieving hard-won success. And if you think that this is a pitfall that's easy to avoid, think again! After all, look at the images we see all the time, on TV, in magazines. "What messages do they give you?" I asked my group during a meeting devoted to body image.

"You're only beautiful if you weigh one hundred and twenty pounds!" a thin, well-spoken woman answered.

"I'm a Latina," a young woman put in. "Latin women have hips. The girls in the magazines have no hips, no thighs. I have to accept that I'm different—that I have curves. I have to work through this, to see that this is who *I* am."

"Does anyone here want to look like Kate Moss?" I asked.

"She looks like she's about to drop dead," someone answered. "Beauty is in the eye of the beholder. If we're here, we're trying. That's all that counts."

We have to stop comparing the way we look with unrealistic models, or even with the way we used to look when we were younger, before we were married, before we had our first child. What do these comparisons accomplish? They become excuses to eat and only distract us. Our job is to climb out of the hole.

I could go on with this list forever. Sometimes you learn how to deal with one factor, only to be pushed into the hole by another. It takes a great deal of time and patience to learn all the varying factors that led you to put on your weight in the first place.

So we're talking about a process of self-discovery, self-knowledge, something that takes time—along with putting into effect very specific techniques, like drinking eight glasses of water a day, like walking up the two floors to the office without taking an elevator. It's a combination of self-examination *and* of developing new habits.

Just a simple habit of never eating standing up can make a world of difference. The streets are full of people eating pizza as they're running to the bus, people with a falafel in one hand, a cellular phone in the other, who haven't discovered the simple process of sitting down, relaxing, eating slowly, savoring every mouthful, and then feeling satisfied. They've had a whole meal, but they're still hungry. Of course they are! They've satisfied their stomachs, but that's all.

During a meeting, one of my group members said, "I remember going over to my parents' house with some groceries for them. It was cold, it was rainy, and when I came in, I looked like a drowned rat. But I didn't eat the cake my mother put out. When she told me to eat something, I told her I had eaten before I came. My father said, 'Have some coffee. Have something to eat. This way you'll feel better. You'll feel nice and warm.'

"There are many times when I've given in, even though my mother's cooking is the worst in the world. When she throws a fish into boiling water, I hate to see it drown. When she takes a roast out of the oven, it looks completely gray. And all my life, she cooked for everyone, and she would make each individual person whatever they liked. Every morning she would take all our requests—and she knows what a terrible cook she is! When the subject comes up, she just laughs. On some level, she knows it's not just about taste; it's about love, it's about memories, it's about one hundred and one things you can't even put into words." People applauded her at the meeting when she was finished—and her story is one I can identify with, too.

The Whys and the Wherefores

I knew a group leader who used to say to her members, "The dictionary defines hunger as a weakened condition due to lack of food." She would stare at the group and narrow her eyes and pound on the table as she asked: "Has anyone in this room ever been hungry?" Enough said.

One of my favorite topics for meetings consists of asking people why they eat and jotting down the answers on the blackboard. In half an hour, the board is always filled with all kinds of reasons, ranging from the rational to the totally crazy, and usually I can identify with each one of them. You eat because you're happy, you eat because you're sad; you eat because you have too much to do, you eat because you have nothing to do. You eat because a holiday is coming, you eat because the holiday has passed and you feel a letdown—and you won't be able to stay on your diet anyway! You eat to reward yourself, you eat to punish yourself.

You eat because it's wintertime, you eat because it's summertime. One of my members said that she eats for the pleasure and satisfaction of eating. Chewing and swallowing. She needs no other reason. Usually, however, the reasons are multilayered and sometimes even self-contradictory.

Can you imagine that one day I decided that my problem had to be a medical one. I didn't eat like a bird—okay, I was ready to admit that fact to myself. But as I looked in the mirror with amazement and horror I asked myself: *Do I really eat so much that I deserve to look like this?* So I went to an endocrinologist and went through a battery of tests, hoping to find something wrong with my metabolism. When the doctor announced I was fine, I was actually disappointed—that's how far gone I was. So what was my response? I ate! I binged! It made me eat more since I realized help wasn't going to come from a pill.

As a young mother, I used to be shipped off to the bungalow colonies in the summer with my children. Do you know what a bungalow colony is? It's where you go to get out of the city. It's a way of getting the kids outdoors. During the week, the wives wear big, loose dresses—smocks, muumuus, *schmattes*. They eat and gossip all day, and at night they gossip and play mah-jongg. I would stay in my bungalow and read, and every night I would make myself a bowl of chocolate icing and eat the whole thing. Four years of that! And those big, loose dresses that covered everything up.

Our husbands arrived on the weekends. I felt like I was in quarantine. To make things worse, apart from the isolation, the other ladies were critical of the way I was raising my children. By the end, I couldn't fit into my weekend outfits, and I was wearing those big, loose dresses seven days a week.

Looking back on my situation now, you might say I had every reason to eat. I was surrounded by critical people, I was out of my own environment, I was bored, unhappy, and lonely. On the other hand, you could turn that around and say I had every reason *not* to eat. That if I had maintained control over my weight and/or forced myself into a more active physical life (swimming, exercising, walking, etc.), I would have been happy.

There was a man in my group who faced a similar situation.

He had divorced his wife, who then moved down to Florida with their teenage son and remarried. The boy was arrested on drug charges and the man had to go to Florida (the stepfather was away on a business trip) and deal with the situation. He said to me, "Rosalie, I was out of town, I didn't have the routine of my job, I was dealing with a crisis that I thought I'd put behind me. I was dealing with my ex-wife . . . my son's drug problem really depressed me. But I kept thinking, *The only thing I have control over is what I put into my mouth*. I didn't give in to bingeing and that fact made me feel much better, especially when I returned."

But all of this is only half the struggle. Because one of the most important aspects of this whole process only begins *after the weight is off!* Most of the time, people pay attention *only* when there is a crisis. The doctor tells you you're eating your way into the grave. You can't fit into any clothes. You have trouble just getting up from a chair. But once you lose the weight, the sense of emergency is over. You're no longer in crisis and it becomes harder and harder to make *yourself* the priority—which is what you have had to do to lose the weight. Nobody drops fifty or sixty pounds without making a major effort, and after the weight is off this effort must continue. You can't just grab whatever's easier to eat—that was the way you put on the pounds to begin with, with junk food and sweets. You have to shop, cook, plan, figure out how much you've eaten that day. You have to exercise, rest when you're tired (instead of eat), talk things out with your spouse or your friends when you're upset (instead of eat), go to the movies, the theater, the library when you're bored (instead of eat)—you have to continue to take the more difficult but more rewarding path.

When the crisis is over, the motivation starts to slip. We become ungrateful, we forget the agony we were in and all we can think of are the pleasures we miss now. We forget how we looked, how we felt, and we complain that a stir fry is no substitute for ice cream. It reminds me of that old joke about a grandmother watching her granddaughter at the beach. A wave comes along and carries the child away from the shore. The grandmother prays—*Dear God, I'll do anything! Anything! Just restore the child to me!*—when all of a sudden, another wave throws the child back on shore. The grandmother runs forward and kisses her and then looks back toward heaven as she says: *She had a hat, you know!* That's human nature! The longer we're on maintenance, the easier it is to forget what it was like before. That's the time to open this book up to the chapter titled *THE LAST STRAW* and compare some of the experiences in it with some of our own. It never hurts to remember where we've come from, to re-examine the reason we wanted to be thin to begin with.

Making A Great Deal: What You Give Up Versus What You Get

At one of my meetings, I asked people to tell me the price they had to pay for being overweight—I asked them to be honest about it, to chalk up the pros and cons, to discuss the rewards and the difficulties of the "thin life." First let's look at some of the cons that people came up with:

- "The truth is, you just get tired of watching what you eat all the time, no matter how motivated you are. That's an inevitable part of the process."
- "It's a commitment, a major decision to be here, to weigh in, to count, etc. Sometimes I think it's worth it, and sometimes— especially when I'm stressed out and want to eat—I don't."
- A lifetime member, a lady whose blood pressure had greatly improved since her weight loss, said: "I have a sign on my refrigerator: *NOTHING TASTES AS GOOD AS BEING THIN FEELS!* One day my son-in-law, who is overweight, looked at it and asked me, 'Ma, do you really believe that?' And do you know what I said to him? 'No!' Because at that moment, I would have given anything to be able to eat the way I used to. So I guess the answer to your question would depend on my mood. But I must believe it more than I didn't believe it, because I'm still thin!"
- "I'm doing the work, but I don't have the rewards—I've been playing with the same five pounds all summer. I can't make a breakthrough."

"Yet," I said to her, "you know what you have to do. In my mind, there's only one question: *What am I willing to do?* I know what I have to do, but am I willing to do it?"

"*You* don't have to worry," someone called out to me.

"That's not true. I'm always in danger of putting on weight again, because I'm a little more relaxed. It's not major weight, that's true, only a pound or so. But I have to pull myself back. I have to tighten up my control again. I used to say: *No! No! No!* Now I say: *No! No! MAYBE!*"

- "I miss the comfort of food—I never took a Valium, I took a chocolate cake. When I was fat, I never had a headache. I miss the reward of as much ice cream as I want. Unlimited chocolate."
- "Staying thin is a lot of work—you have to worry about having the right food ready all the time. That means shopping, preparing, figuring."
- "For me, the hardest part is the self-denial. I know I'm allowed to eat my favorite foods but I don't have enough control to eat them without going overboard. So I have to give up all the foods I love."
- "It's a constant choice—I'm sick of the struggle."
- "Time! That's my number one gripe. It takes so long to think salad, fish, to weigh and measure and all that. A chocolate bar takes a split second to unwrap."
- "It takes a long time to lose weight. You work and you work at it, and you don't see the results—or at least you don't see them for a long while. When I work, I want to get the rewards right away."
- "It's not natural—we always have to make an effort."
- "The healthier, the better the food is, the more it costs."
- "You're always refusing people—at home, at work, you're always saying 'No' to foods you'd love to eat and which people keep pushing on you."

I think of these *cons* as the price tag of what it costs to be thin. It's good to have a realistic idea of just what the struggle entails, because then you are prepared for what you will encounter. Now for the *pros,* which are all-too-often forgotten when the impulse to eat strikes:

- "When I'm eating in a controlled way, I feel good. Not only healthier, but more optimistic about life."
- "I have more self-confidence. I'm not afraid to go out in public."
- "I like looking good."
- "I feel younger."
- "I feel sexier—and that's always good for my sex life. My husband picks up on it right away."
- "I have more energy."
- "I think it will enable me to live longer. I want to see my grandchildren grow up."
- "I hate being out of control."
- "I want to fit into my clothes."
- "For me, it's not clouding my thinking with food. Instead of rushing to eat chocolate, now I think about the way I'm feeling. If I'm feeling bad, I examine my feelings."
- "If you ask me," a mother of three said, "a major reason I decided to lose weight was because I love to dance, but I can't go on as long as I used to. Because of my weight, I start huffing and puffing after ten minutes on the dance floor. And now that I said I would lose the weight, I feel as if I have to. My kids watch me. If I skip a meeting they say to me, 'You're not quitting, are you? You're not giving up?' I don't want to set them a bad example."
- "No matter what good things are going on in my life, there's a low level of depression when I'm fat. I'm never really happy when I know I'm carrying an extra fifty or sixty pounds. And once I start losing, I feel this depression lift."
- "I feel terrible when I have extra weight on my joints."
- "When I'm in control of my weight, it carries over into other areas of my life."
- "I'm more assertive when I'm thin. I stand up for myself more."

The benefits of weight loss are many, from a healthier life to a more fulfilling one. It is important to keep them in mind, because having a clear sense of our goals and achievements helps us fight off the impulse to quit, to binge, to go back to our old eating patterns when difficulties arise, as they inevitably must.

As one member, a very intelligent woman who'd lost close to seventy pounds, put it: "If you're upset and tell yourself that you will only eat until a particular problem is solved, then another problem comes along right afterwards. There will always be something—always some problem, some bill, some pressure. And you know what I've found? In six months or so, most of the problems resolve themselves one way or another—so what's the use of worrying about them, of eating ourselves up alive? What good does it do to face life fat?"

"Yes," a nurse in the group added, "I've just 'allowed myself' to go off the program for three days because I was constantly on call. But what did I accomplish by putting my eating needs on the back burner? At first I thought I wouldn't exercise, since I didn't have the time. But that had a ripple effect. I stopped writing down what I ate and ended up eating a box of chocolates—and I have a family history of diabetes."

"You have to learn that nothing can take priority over your own needs," I said, "because there will always be a reason to start losing control."

"But doesn't it get easier after so many years?" a new member asked me.

"I know you'd like me to say it does—but the answer to that one is 'sometimes'. I can coast along for months without a struggle and then, suddenly, the temptation begins again. I have a voracious sweet tooth and *sometimes* what I wouldn't do to be able to satisfy it in the old way! *Sometimes* it almost feels as if I were back where I started from—only with a lot more awareness and many techniques at my disposal.

"That's why even now, even after twenty-two years of keeping my weight off, I respect my boundaries. I know what puts me at risk. For example, before I walk out of my door in the morning, I must know exactly what I'm going to eat and I must have it with me. Or, to give another example, after a party or a holiday, the extra food must be out of my house; it must all be gone. The struggle never ends. Even now, after twenty-two years, when a problem arises, I have to keep telling myself: *There's no way you're going to get fat over this!* I have to make sure that my needs for free time or relaxation aren't pushed aside. If they are, I'll end up satisfying those needs in the fridge or at the bakery. Slowly, people have gotten used to who I am now: I don't bake anymore. I'm willing to help people, to *put out* for them, but only within the limits I've established. And so on—I've made a lot of changes.

"Of course it was easier to turn to food as a cure-all! It was easier in the short run, but the long-term price was too high! It's a terrible, desperate way of life. I've known both ways, and for all the effort my new life costs, it was worth it." That answer summed up where I was—and where I'd come from.

For me, the following story explains it all.

An ant and an elephant got married—so the story goes. The morning after the honeymoon, the elephant dropped dead. And there's the ant standing next to the huge carcass, crying and screaming hysterically: "One night of ecstasy, and now I have to spend the rest of my life digging a grave."

The moment of ecstasy might be ice cream, chocolate cake, fried chicken—whatever. It's the moment when we flee from whatever's bothering us and escape into a world of pleasure. But then comes the lifetime of trying to "bury" the consequences and we're forced to ask ourselves, *Was it worth it?* For those struggling to free themselves of their addiction to food, the answer to this question is a loud and clear NO! It is to them that I dedicate this book.

CHAPTER TWO

The Last Straw

"I'm through lying to myself. From now on, denial—de Nile—
is a river in Egypt."

—Rosalie Kaufman, Group Leader

"There are no nouveau fat in this room."

—A member

Drop a grain of sand into an oyster and the irritation will form
a pearl. It's the same process with us—what makes us change?
Something has to happen that makes the pain of being overweight
greater than the pleasure of eating what we want. At the time, this
experience might seem humiliating or shattering, but the truth is
that if we know how to *make use of it*, it can become a wake-up
call that empowers us, enabling us to take charge of our lives.

Sometimes people can be so cruel! There's a young husband
and wife team—I would say both of them are in their late twenties—who attend one of my meetings. The wife is beautiful and
never had a weight problem until recently. When she discovered
that she'd put on around fifteen pounds, she decided to join her
husband at the meetings—his problem was more long-standing
and serious. He'd lost over one hundred pounds at one point in
his life and then gained them all back. When his wife started
showing up with him, he had taken off about forty pounds and
was struggling with sixty-odd pounds. Heavy or not, he's a very
lively, intelligent, warm, kind person—someone who brightens up
the day when he enters the room. And yet people have actually

come up to his wife and said, *What are you doing with him?* referring to his being overweight.

"The ironic part of it is that before she told me that, I was just about to quit," he said. "But after I heard that, nothing could stop me. The one thought that went through my head was, *They'll see.*"

His wife told me confidentially, "Rosalie, I love him any way he is. But I don't want to keep reassuring him of that because I want him to change for his own sake. Diabetes runs in his family and he's putting himself at high risk. So I let him know what people were saying—and I'm glad to say it had a good effect."

In my case, I heard it from the horse's mouth. I remember spending hours getting ready to attend a large charity fund-raiser with my husband. I especially wanted to look good because my husband was making a speech and I was sitting next to him on the dais. The only trouble was that I was fifty pounds overweight while my husband is the kind of a man who never gains a pound. If he still had the suit he'd worn at our wedding, it would fit him. We made an odd couple, with him so trim and fit and me so large— I must have known this but I didn't let myself really know it until a "friend" whispered in a voice loud enough for all to hear, "She looks like his mother." It's true that my weight made me look much older, but I didn't have to be made to realize it that way— just because I was fat didn't mean I was deaf. But instead of just feeling sorry for myself, my friend's words made me angry. *They'll see!* I decided and, having given up without even realizing it, I took a deep breath and began the struggle once again. My friend's cruelty was my last straw or, I should say, *one of them,* because I needed to be prodded into action again and again until I achieved success.

And it's not just me; I've heard countless stories like this because overweight people inevitably undergo a lot of pain and humiliation in our society. We might not agree with it, but that's how it is. A fact of life. And sometimes that cruelty affects not only ourselves, but those we love. A young mother in one of my groups noticed that her son regularly came home from school bruised and scratched. Since he wasn't an angry child, she had a long talk with him and he finally admitted why he was getting into fights: other kids at school were calling her names on account of her weight.

That was enough to do it for her—she went on the program and has kept forty pounds off to this day. My daughter dated a young man whose mother was morbidly obese, over four hundred pounds. He said that he'd never thought about it much until he went to kindergarten and when she came to school the kids made fun of her.

The pain cuts across all classes, all ethnic groups. An environmental lawyer who has been a group member for the last five years shared with us the moment that stopped her in her tracks. She was being honored for her hard work raising money to maintain an upstate wildlife preserve; at the awards dinner, she was seated next to a slim, well-dressed female reporter. The contrast between them was striking—she knew she didn't look good in the black sack she'd worn to cover up the pounds; she felt dowdy and heavy to begin with, but her feelings were intensified when the dessert showed up. The reporter—maybe being malicious, maybe just being unconsciously cruel—pushed her dessert toward the lawyer and asked loud enough for others to hear, "Would you like mine, too?" The evening, which should have been one of pride and triumph for her, turned sour. At that moment she vowed, *I'll never eat chocolate again!* (her favorite binge food) and while the truth is that she has eaten chocolate many times since—*never* and *always* are words for lovers, not Weight Watchers®!—she has kept off almost sixty pounds since that awards dinner. She wrote those words over her fridge and made them her slogan, so that every time she was tempted, she would mutter under her breath: *Would you like mine, too?* as a way of keeping the memory alive.

Sometimes the cruelty is inflicted unconsciously. One of my group members told me that she went into a store to buy some summer clothes and before she could ask the clerk for what she wanted, she was told: *Oh no, we don't have anything in your size.* "She didn't ask me what my size was," the woman said. "She didn't measure me. She just took one look and knew."

I'm sure the clerk didn't mean to inflict pain: she was just thoughtless. The same thing happened to another member, a wonderful woman who takes care of both her elderly parents and her husband's invalid mother. She was at her niece's wedding, and was standing at the buffet waiting to be served. When the waitress handed her a plate of Chinese food, another waitress, also working at the buffet, said: *That won't be enough for her. Put some more on the plate.* "Her tone was kind, Rosalie," she said. "She wasn't trying to insult me. Just the opposite. But when I heard those words, I felt like going through the floor. I just took the plate and slunk away. But I vowed then and there to change."

In her case, the sting came from another's thoughtlessness, but it doesn't have to. Just last week, a woman from England put it simply and poignantly at one of my meetings: "It grieves me that I can no longer wear my wedding ring," she said. She had been going along trying to ignore what was happening to her body, but it was impossible to ignore her wedding ring. It had too much significance for her—her husband was very poor when he'd bought it; it had been the result of much sacrifice and much love. And now taking it off was like parting with a piece of her history. It forced her to take a long look at what was happening: was that the route she really wanted to go?

Self-Image: Fantasy Versus Reality

Sometimes a physical problem is the wake-up call. A very large woman described to us what had brought her to Weight Watchers® during her first meeting. She is middle-aged with beautiful features, a woman who could be stunning and who knows how to dress— elegant clothes, fine jewelry, the works. With a tremor in her voice, she said: "I went to a doctor and he told me: 'If you lose one hundred pounds your knees won't hurt any more.'

"Who is he talking to? That's what I couldn't figure out," she said with *such* pain in her voice. "I was in a state of shock. I couldn't believe I'd let myself put on one hundred pounds. I always dressed right, always took care of myself. To hear this all of a sudden was just too much for me."

The image she had of herself no longer matched the reality. And so something had to happen. In this case, the meeting with the doctor brought the reality home and started her on the path to rejoining her own inner image. She used the shock so constructively, in fact, that not only did she get rid of the pain in her knees, but she became one of the most striking women I have ever seen.

What would have happened without that visit to the doctor? You would think it wouldn't be possible to gain a hundred pounds and not really be aware of it—but it is. The pounds creep up; you get used to yourself at one size, then a size larger becomes the norm, and then the next. It takes a long time for someone who is thin to realize they have gotten heavy or for someone who is heavy to realize they have become obese. A marriage where eating is loving, going away to school for the first time without Mama's cooking—any number of changes can affect a person's eating pattern and then the pounds creep up.

"I shouldn't be here," a physical therapist said in one of my groups, "since I see what happens to overweight people all the time in the hospital. We have trouble lifting them—it takes three or four of us sometimes. We have to measure them for special wheelchairs. We have problems getting them through the doors. Therapists sometimes groan when they get assigned to heavy patients, since it's such hard work. But here I am with twenty extra pounds and gaining more weight every day. I came to stop myself."

"What got you motivated?" I asked her. "Was it fear?"

"I didn't even realize how I'd let myself go," she answered, "until a fellow worker made a joke at my expense. I won't say what it was. At first I thought she was talking about one of the patients, but when I realized *I* was the person she meant, I had to sit down to take it in. I just never realized what was happening."

"The same was true of me," a young woman who worked in a nursing home said. "When I attended my brother's wedding, I thought I looked gorgeous. But when we sat down to watch the videos, I kept thinking: *Who is that elephant in purple chiffon?*" Later, she showed me a photo and the dress was one of what I call our "disguises": outfits which we *think* make us look great—large, loose, billowing creations that are supposed to cover a multitude of sins but in reality only make us look worse. This woman is intelligent, capable, entrusted with responsibility—but when it came to seeing a simple fact about herself, she was blind until that wedding. While she was able to take care of so many others, she had given up when it came to taking care of herself. The changes she has undergone in the last two years are truly remarkable. But she needed something to force her to take action.

Sometimes the motivation is very specific. A young woman who was about twenty-five pounds overweight came up to me after her first meeting to ask some questions about the program and ended up talking about what had brought her to Weight Watchers®. "I dated a guy I liked last year," she said. "It wasn't all that serious, but we had a good rapport. We were taking the same classes—we're both science majors—and had a lot in common. But I think the reason we hit it off was because I had a lot of self-confidence then. I was looking good—I'd gotten down to a size eight, and I was wearing sexy clothes and had a new hairdo, so I found it easy to start up a conversation with him.

"The trouble was that I lost the weight with diet pills and when I had to stop taking the pills (they were making me very nervous), I began regaining it. He went back to California over the summer and when he saw me this fall, I could see he was shocked. He didn't say anything about my weight, but I know how different I looked. Anyway, he hasn't asked me out again and now I want to try again, only without the pills."

I've heard so many stories like that: people lose the weight because they want a relationship, which is natural enough. Wanting a relationship isn't a bad way *to get started*. At some point, though, the process has to become internalized—they have to want to lose weight for themselves as well, or else it won't last. It won't become a part of their life. When problems arise in the relationship or they are disappointed, they'll go back to their old style of eating.

A middle-aged widow in one of my groups wouldn't consider even meeting anyone until she took off her weight. "I'd be too embarrassed," she said to me privately after one of the meetings. "It's so important for me to lose weight, but I keep bingeing. I can't understand it." My guess is that her anxiety about dating again only made it harder for her to face her weight issues. It was too much pressure.

"I moved from LA to New York when my husband got trans-ferred and I put on about ten pounds," a young wife said during a meeting. "I was overweight to begin with, but those extra ten pounds put me over the limit, although I didn't realize it right away. I had a hard time getting used to the winter, the new way of life here, and to being so far away from all of my family and my good friends. In LA I used to go out walking every morning, but once the cold weather started here, forget it. It was all I could do to get out of bed."

"Yes," I said, "a move is a major change in life which can take a long time to absorb."

"The bottom line was that I didn't think of myself as being *so* overweight. My mind was on other things, anyway. Until one day, I was leaving for work when I heard the young boy a few houses down say to a UPS delivery man: "No, this isn't for us. It's for that fat lady over there." He didn't mean it maliciously—he was only a kid. But I'd become *that fat lady*. It made me realize what had happened to me."

There are as many last straws as there are people—a mother notices that she can no longer take care of her young children when she takes them to the park. She is only twenty-seven but if her two-year-old needs to be picked up or her four-year-old needs to be chased after, she does not have the breath or the stamina.

A very overweight woman breaks her leg and has to be carried to an ambulance by a team of struggling volunteers. There is no way she can hide from the fact that five healthy men have trouble moving her. A businesswoman traveling in Eastern Europe is humiliated when a flight on a small plane is delayed because her seat belt doesn't fit. "*Mortified* doesn't even begin to describe how I felt. There were ten people on that flight and they all turned and stared at me while the stewardess struggled with my belt! Finally they found extenders for the belt, but I couldn't look anyone in the eye for that whole flight."

The list is endless.

Let's Tie A String Around Our Finger!

The truth of the matter is, why we get motivated is directly related to our *continued* motivation. It's important to keep this in mind for this chapter is not only about beginnings; just the opposite, these last straws are even more important later on in the process. In the beginning, overweight people are often very motivated— they've suffered any number of embarrassing moments and humiliations. They are dying to change and in most cases are afraid of what's happening to them: the numbers keep going up and up and up, so they take themselves in hand and go on a program of sane eating. But time goes by and then—it's not that they forget, but they need to recapture the initial motivation given to them by the last straw. They need to *feel* what they felt in the beginning to keep going.

That's what happened to a woman I'll call my Trucking Lady. She was a tough, seasoned businesswoman who'd built up a large company all on her own, dealing in a man's world. Her husband helped her, but she was the boss. He specialized in disappearing acts. He was the kind of man who was at the racetrack the day she gave birth—an event which was also her *last straw:*

"I always had hard labors. Fifteen hours or so," she said. "With my last one, I was in the late stages. I couldn't move a muscle and was in agony when they decided to give me an epidural, so they had to move me. The nurse, a young blonde who I guess a lot of people would have called pretty, was flirting with the doctor and when they started to move me, she said to him, 'I hope you've had your Cheerios this morning.' People say you forget what happens in labor, but even now, twenty-two years later, every word that bitch said is fresh in my mind. I'm used to being on top of things, but at that moment I felt like shit. You have no way to defend yourself when you're in that state, and here I was, being reminded of what my body looked like to strangers. It was a dumb joke at my expense which made me vow that I'd never overeat again. Everyone who's fat like I was fat has gone through things like that."

If you think this woman got off the labor table and never binged again, you're wrong. To add to her obstacles, of course, was the weight she'd put on during pregnancy and the extra difficulty of getting it off. But I've had women come in wanting to lose the thirty or forty pounds they've put on while they were pregnant and—give me a break!—the kid is seventeen. Women *have been known* to give birth and lose weight afterwards; it's harder, but it can be done.

In the case of my trucking lady, though, she ended up never losing more than five pounds. Plus she regained *thirteen* of those five pounds when I last met her—which wasn't at a Weight Watchers® meeting, by the way—because she gave up. She is still tortured by her weight, but is unable to do anything about it. At least for the present. Maybe some day in the future she'll remember how she felt on that labor table, pick herself up, and start again.

Everything depends on a person's frame of mind. Sometimes we can look at a photo and say, "Boy, do I look fat *in that picture—*" and not connect the way we look in *that picture* with reality. We deny it. The camera caught us at a bad angle. *(Yeah! Like bending over!)* The film was overexposed. *(Right! And maybe our derrière was, too!)*

Other times, we see the picture clearly and we get to work on ourselves. The point is that maybe we have to be ready for the last straw in order for it to *become* the last straw. In that receptive frame of mind, anything can trigger our resolve. For example, there was a woman I'll call my Pizza Girl because she would regularly telephone the local pizzeria and order an extra large pie for herself with double cheese and all the trimmings. Whenever the delivery man came to the door, she used to pretend that the pizza wasn't just for her and call back into her empty apartment, "Honey, it's here!" or "Chow time!"

But one day, she heard herself calling back into that empty apartment and thought: *This is pathetic! This is not the way I want to live my life.* For her that moment was a last straw—and she made it work. She saw herself clearly. And she used that insight to get back on track quickly—without doing any more damage.

Sometimes it's an accumulation of small incidents that combine into a wake-up call. This happened to one of my group members whose operative thought for many years was: *Who cares if I'm a fat old lady?* But then she found herself out walking with friends and more and more often she couldn't keep up. She'd have people in the house and by eleven-thirty PM she could hardly wait for them to leave so she could get undressed and get into the sack she wore around the house. When she walked in the street she looked away so she did not see herself in store windows.

For me, *one* of my last straws—and, as I said, I needed several—was clothing. I could lie to myself about how I looked in photos, I could explain away my sluggishness and shortness of breath when I walked up the stairs, but there was no way I could fit into clothes that once fit me.

I remember vividly when sportswear became fashionable. Women started wearing skirts and tops and jackets instead of dresses, and at A&S, I tried on a top that said ONE SIZE FITS ALL, but guess what? It didn't.

And I went home and ate. I had money in my wallet that I wanted to spend because I wanted to look good but there was nothing I could buy. There was no FORGOTTEN WOMAN or CHARISMA, no fashionable clothes for overweight women. You went to Lane Bryant or Roaman's and you bought a polyester muumuu in various floral prints. I was not ready to move into a floral printed muumuu at the age of thirty-five. Besides which, I had eaten my way through the sizes in the regular store and I could see myself starting at the smallest size in one of those other stores and eating my way up the range.

Clothes don't lie, but there are also life situations which force us to realize that things have gone too far. It can be something as simple as the fact that we have to lie down on a bed to zip up our pants. Or it can be as dramatic as seeing ourselves through someone else's eyes. A woman I'll call The Desperado told a story I've heard many times over—the details are always different, but the point is always the same.

In the middle of a meeting that was supposed to be about exercise, she went off on an emotional tangent. I suppose she felt so bad that she just had to tell somebody about it. And everybody responded—because everybody had been there themselves. I had asked the question, *What are we willing to do to be thin?*, expecting to hear people talk about joining gyms or buying exercise machines.

She groaned, "Oh, not *that* again! My husband gives me that every day: 'Some wives would do anything for their husbands and you won't even give up your food for me.'"

"Tell him to shove it," one of my more refined members advised.

"Every time my boyfriend gets on my case I go straight to the fridge," another woman added.

"What do they know? Just because everybody overeats from time to time, they all think they're experts," an older woman said with feeling.

"Okay," I said and held up my hands. "So we've determined that they're idiots, they're fools, and that we deserve everything on our plates and more. Let's get back to the question: *What are you willing to do to change?*"

"At this point I'm so desperate," one very large woman said, "that I'll do anything! Anything at all!"

"Except give up your food!" The Desperado added and laughed bitterly.

"That's your husband speaking, I bet," I said, trying to get her to calm down and talk it out.

"The problem is, he's right. Oh, not about me loving my food more than I love him. I do love him. But one thing has nothing to do with the other and he just can't see that."

"Is that really true?" a successful woman who was on maintenance asked. "If you really love someone and know something is important to him, maybe you'd change for his sake."

"Why can't *he* just love *her* the way she is without making her turn herself inside out for him?" the older woman asked.

"The truth is, we can't change for anyone else. We can only change if *we* want to," I put in.

"But I *do* want to change!" she said. "I'm not happy being out of control. Forget the way I look! I'm not happy running around eating everything in sight."

"So what's the problem? I don't see it," the older woman asked. "Lose the weight and then both of you will be happy."

"I don't know. I just can't," she said.

"You mean you haven't—*so far,*" I said.

"How do you expect her to lose with her husband breathing down her neck? He thinks he's helping her but he's not. He's only pressuring her."

"But you know what?" The Desperado said. "Without him, I wouldn't have even tried. We used to have—we still have—a lot of fights about how fat I was getting and I'd always promise never to binge again and then end up breaking my promise. But one day it got really bad. We had just finished eating breakfast together— bagels, eggs, the works. That was part of our new plan: I was supposed to eat like a 'normal person' and that would stop me from bingeing. But the minute he left the house for work, I went straight to the fridge, looking like a scavenger for whatever I could find. There happened to be some of General Tsao's Famous Chicken we'd ordered in from a Chinese take-out place the night before. I'd cleaned my plate but there was plenty left over from my husband, his brother and my sister-in-law, all 'naturally thin' people."

"I'll bet that got to you," someone remarked. "It always gets to me."

"I guess it did—the idea of all that food going to waste—"

"People are starving in China, right?" another lady added. "It's a sin to waste food!"

"So anyway, there I was at eight-thirty in the morning with a feast of cold Chinese food spread out over the kitchen table—I didn't even wait to heat it up—when my husband came back for something he forgot. If he'd walked in on me and another man, I couldn't have been more horrified. I tried to act normal but he just stood there looking at me as if I was crazy. And that's when I decided to weigh in, to join up, the whole bit."

"So what you're saying is that if he hadn't come home, you wouldn't have felt bad?" the older woman asked.

"I guess I wouldn't have been forced to see how out of control things had gotten. I wouldn't have let myself think about it."

"But did you join for him or for yourself? That's still the question," the successful woman said.

"To be honest, I really don't know. But I know that now, after being here for three months, I come here because I want to come. I come for myself."

"I think that's great," I said and there was scattered applause around the room. "But I still say your husband should back off now. You can explain to him that he helped you in the beginning, but that if he really wants to help you, he'll let you fight this one out yourself."

This woman did very well for about six months, losing almost twenty-five pounds to her delight and the delight of her husband who, seeing her seriousness, had agreed to keep out of it. But then the weight loss stopped for a week and the next week she was up two pounds and the week after that, one pound more.

"What's happening to me?" she asked, coming up to me before a meeting. "I don't understand what's gone wrong." And after listening to her describe her week, I diagnosed a case of what I call 'mid-diet slump.' Those of us who have stuck with a program for any length of time know how it happens—we see that the initial bloat has come off and the weight loss is slowing down; "friends" are telling us that we look great and that we shouldn't lose any more (maybe something we've been secretly telling ourselves). Perhaps we've lost twenty or thirty pounds and by now we aren't willing to take the time to find or prepare interesting foods. We fall into a rut and end up eating the same meal again and again so we get bored and disgusted. It's not as if we wake up one morning and say, *I'm going to start eating now*. It's usually a slow process of erosion.

Working at Inspiration

The woman had come a long way from the day her husband caught her with the Chinese food. She'd taken so many positive steps toward success: her muscle-tone was returning, her body was beginning to regain its shape, she'd bought new clothes, her relationship with her husband had improved. "Try to focus on where you've come from," I told her. "Build on your success."

Many times we take our hard-won successes for granted at this mid-point and only think of how much more weight we have to lose. She needed to find some new activity that would lift her out of the doldrums—maybe joining a dance class or going to movies or the theater would do it for her. Maybe she could pamper herself with a massage or a facial and manicure. If she could just hang on and get through this difficult period, she had every possibility of reaching her goal.

She agreed and tried, but when she came in the next week she was up half a pound and felt discouraged.

"What would you have done in the old days when you felt the way you do now?" I asked her.

"I would have binged nonstop," she answered without a moment's hesitation.

"And how much do you think you would have put on? Five pounds, ten?"

She nodded.

"Well, a half-pound gain represents success for you at this point. First you gained two pounds, then you gained one pound—now it's only a half pound. You're putting the brakes on. You can get rid of that half pound in a single week! You've proven that you can do it—you've lost twenty-five pounds and have kept off twenty-two and a half of those twenty-five. That's the way to think—focus on what you've kept off, not on the little bit you've gained back. Now make up your mind, because it's up to you. The decision is in your hands and you can do it."

She struggled through the next month, losing a pound here, gaining a pound there. But finally, at the end of that month she regained control and started to lose steadily. What had upset her during that month is hard to say. Sometimes you just reach a point where you resist change—who knows?

"I work in Special Ed," said a young woman who's been in my group for about a year, "and although I love my job, it's a very difficult one. I come home at the end of the day so burned out that the only thing that recharges me is a fudge sundae or a half gallon of ice cream—*before* I start dinner. But this year, when I went to the doctor for a routine checkup, she sat me down and did something that made me realize what I was doing to myself. She just pulled out my chart and wrote down my weight on a piece of paper, along with the year. She started five years back and then continued on into the future, using my steady rate of gain to predict where I was going. That's all she had to do. She didn't say another word, but I went to Weight Watchers® the next day."

This young woman is one of the lucky ones—usually people don't think about their health until they lose it. But she saw that there had to be another way.

"I still come home stressed," she said, "but now I try to work it off on an exercise machine. I used to think that at the end of a hard day, it would be too difficult. But the strange thing is, it gets my blood racing, it gives me more energy instead of taking it away, and I find I enjoy the evening more after a workout. I only hope it keeps up."

Sometimes loving wives will join Weight Watchers because of their husbands, or vice versa, and then they get motivated on their own account. One woman who did this continued on even after her husband dropped out: "I discovered that I felt better and looked better with my eating under control. I just hope I can get my husband to come back," she said. "I've changed the way I cook and I encourage him to join me for walks, but there's just so much you can do."

"In the long run, a person's fate is in their own hands." I said.

Over the years, I've had people join along with young children as a way of licking the problem together. "What mobilized me was seeing my daughter following in my footsteps," said a mother in her mid-thirties with two daughters, the younger one very chubby. "It's bad enough that I've suffered with my weight all my life. I didn't want that for her, too, so I decided to take action." And she was right, of course, because children learn from our example.

When it comes to dealing with young children—in this case her daughter was ten—there are specific steps you can take that will make a difference. I advise parents not to put too much pressure on the child. At the dinner table, don't say to them, "This is for you and this is not for *you*"—they must not be made to feel different from their brothers and sisters. You can subtly oversee portion size and encourage physical activity without making it into a strict regimen. I tell mothers to have healthy snack foods in the house and to dress them well—good body image is important for children, especially since other kids tend to be cruel. Do whatever you can to bolster their self-image. I know an overweight girl of about eleven in my neighborhood who is effervescent, has a wonderful personality and a beautiful face. I tell her when the other girls make fun of her it is because they are jealous. "Sooner or later," I said to her, "you will take off the weight. But they will never have what you do!" My reward was a big smile, a hug, and a kiss.

So many times desperate people have come up to me—not only at Weight Watchers®, but also in social situations—and asked, "Rosalie, how can I begin?" And I tell them: "Just begin!" Of course, it would help them to learn about food, to learn techniques, to start exercising, but the fact that they're asking the question shows that they've overcome the greatest obstacle—despair.

At that moment they're inspired. They're disgusted with what bingeing has done to their lives and are ready to begin. It's after they've been working seriously on their weight for a number of weeks or even months that they need to remember how they felt at the beginning and rekindle their initial motivation. It's often said that it's an ill wind that blows no good—there's some good mixed in with every bad experience. Why not take the humiliation and pain and turn them into inspiration and the beginning of a new life?

CHAPTER THREE

How-To—Who Says You Can't Have It All?

The Journey of 1,000 Miles Begins With A Single Step
—Found in a Chinese Fortune Cookie (30 calories)

Some people think of discipline as a kind of chore. For me it's the wings that set me free to fly.
—Julie Andrews

"Violins were playing," a woman in my group sighed—I'll call her The Wedding Guest. "A white piano was on a little island in the middle of a fountain—the music, the splashing of the water, the colored lights, the thick carpets—everybody was waiting for the wedding couple to emerge when all of a sudden my mother pulled me to one side, pointed to a side room where the smorgasbord was about to open up, and whispered: *Go on, eat something! Daddy gave them a hundred dollars!* So what did she want? To make the money back? If I ate a hundred and fifty dollars worth of stuffed cabbage, Chinese food, and *kishka,* would that make her happy? But I was only a kid then, I was sixteen, so I went and ate. That's the kind of attitude I grew up with—never waste a morsel of food, eat everything in sight—you know the kind of mentality. I still have to fight that when I go out even though it's so many years later," she said with frustration.

How-To means techniques, strategies, knowing what problems are facing you so you can make a plan in advance. It means, for example, pushing away the bread basket in a restaurant when you sit down to order. You can eat a whole day's worth of bread—

make that a month's worth—without realizing it, just munching away on rolls and crackers as you look over the menu. Remember (although you won't read this in any medical book), the hand and the mouth have a life and a mind of their own! It means knowing your food lists inside and out so you can estimate at a glance how much you're eating. It means studying the food lists! Learning about food! Taking the time to avoid mistakes!

One woman in my group was amazed to learn that pasta was counted as a bread. "What did you think it was?" somebody asked her.

"I don't know," she shrugged. "I just thought it was a healthy food I could eat without worrying."

Someone else convinced herself that nuts were a fruit! Of course these people were bound to gain weight no matter how hard they tried not to.

How-To means drinking water before you start a meal, or learning about low calorie ways to have the food prepared—learning how to prepare steamed, sautéed marinated vegetables or fish at home or asking for the food to be prepared this way in a restaurant instead of ordering fried food. It means looking for words like *grilled* or *poached* or *roasted* on the menu, and cooking this way at home.

"You complain about eating out," I told The Wedding Guest, "but once you have the right techniques down on a day-to-day basis, eating out can be a cinch, something you look forward to. Especially if you've been keeping a record of what you're eating, and have enough leftover calories to fit into your food budget, you can order so many delicious—"

"All right, all right, I know that," The Wedding Guest interrupted me impatiently. "But what am I going to do about the voice in my head that makes me clean my plate?"

"Any ideas?" I turned to the group.

"Well, for me this problem comes up all the time and not just when I'm eating out. If I make a casserole for my family and somebody's not hungry, I can't just put it in the fridge like a normal person and forget about it. I clear the table and begin washing the dishes and the casserole is sitting there. And I'll find myself going back to it and taking a nibble here and a nibble there and before

I know it, it's finished. So I've learned to throw it out right away—even though I was raised NEVER to throw anything out. You know the old routine—people are starving. But it's more of a sin to throw it *in*—to me, I mean—than to throw it *out*. How does it help the starving people if I get fat? If I feel bad, I can give a contribution to charity—I don't have to become a human vacuum cleaner after every meal."

"All right, even though her problem is getting her money's worth—the answer is the same. You have to change the way you look at things and *after that* the way you eat changes," I said, turning to The Wedding Guest. "Many people, though, don't even realize what they're doing or why. They just sit down and automatically finish up whatever's put in front of them. But you've begun to think about why you're doing what you do and that's a good beginning. You know what you're up against. So you've made progress that you can build on since you've thought your behavior through."

Muhammad Ali once said: "The fight is won or lost far away from witnesses behind the lines, in the gym and out there on the road, long before I dance under those lights." Think of weight loss as being in the boxing ring; you have to prepare before you get into the ring if you want to win the match.

One of the winning techniques is getting to the point where you can leave food that you've paid for in restaurants, are given at parties, or have prepared at home. It sounds simple—but it's crucial. In fact, when Wedding Guest told her story, heads around the room began to nod. Many people had the same problem.

A woman in a black jumper cut like a maternity dress spoke up in a gruff, almost angry voice. "Yes, what she's saying is true. I haven't been to a wedding since I was a kid, but I go out to restaurants a lot—I hate to cook—and guess what I finally learned? Are you ready for this? You *can* leave something on your plate!"

Everybody laughed.

"For some people, elegance means the Gucci handbag or the Prada shoes or the Armani suit," I said. "For me it was leaving food on the plate. The first time I did it, I thought fireworks should go off."

"Forget it!" said a woman I'll call Loves To Eat Out. "If I'm paying for it, I'm not throwing it out! But I've learned that doesn't mean I have to eat it all at one sitting, either. The other night my husband and I went to a very special dinner at the Waldorf-Astoria and he was very embarrassed when I asked for a doggie bag. He thought it just wasn't done at a place like the Waldorf. But look at this!" she said, holding up a black velvet bag, a drawstring pouch with the letters W.A. on it in gold. It was so nice that if those were her initials she could have used it for an evening bag. "Without that," she went on, "I never could have left such a delicious mean *unfinished*. And the doggie bag was no big deal. *You see, I told my husband, they wouldn't have these unless a lot of people asked for them, even here!*"

"I feel the same way," a petite, middle-aged lady said. "I'm in my fifties and my son is in his twenties. He's a large man and I'm on the short side. But when we go out to eat, they bring out the same size portions for both of us. Now there's no way I need to eat as much as he does—why should the chef be the one to decide how many calories I take in? The new me has decided if the food is really good, really special, I get a doggie bag—but otherwise I've trained myself to let it go! It's just a matter of habit. Once you've broken out of this compulsion, you're better off. You can pay attention to the way you feel instead of just eating whatever's put in front of you."

Another technique that helps in our boxing match is learning to be assertive when you eat out, learning to insist that your needs are met. "I have a big problem when I go to a restaurant," said a very large woman with a thick Russian accent—I'll call her Garbo. She had joined our group recently and had been making remarkable progress during her first few weeks. "Sometimes they don't understand me and the waiter brings the wrong thing. The salad has oil or the pasta is covered with cheese."

"Maybe the waiter's reading your mind?" someone called out.

"Oh, you don't have to be foreign for them to screw up the order," a schoolteacher said. "I like to be at work early, so instead of making breakfast at home, I go into a coffee shop across the street from my school. When I started going on this program, I began asking them for one scrambled egg but they brought me two. So I said to the manager: *Look, I'll be coming in here every day for breakfast. If you want my business, please make sure I don't have to argue with the waiter every time.* And you know what? It never happened again."

"I did the same thing at a local deli," another woman said. "I told them I didn't want the usual sandwich they made—I wanted four ounces of meat and no more. The waiter didn't listen, and not only that, but when he put the plate in front of me and I complained, he had the nerve to say: *Why don't you just put it on the side?* Of course I didn't want it on the side—I'd end up eating it. So I said, *Are you interested in your tip?* That was enough—he shut up and redid the order. At one point, I never would have insisted—but I've learned it's better to speak up and make it their problem than keep silent and watch the numbers go up."

"Usually people are very happy to help you out at restaurants, especially good restaurants—they want you to come back," I said.

"Listen, when low calorie bread first came out—you know, it's only forty calories a slice—I brought it into a restaurant where I had lunch every week with my friends," a woman who'd been silent until then said. "I'd been attending meetings at a different group and the leader gave me the idea. My friends felt too embarrassed to ask, so they made me the one to give the waiter the bread and ask him to make up our sandwiches with it. I don't know what we thought he'd do—throw us out?—but it was no big deal. He said that as long as we paid the same price, it was all right with him. And you know what? We did that every week afterwards so that when we forgot one week, *he* asked us: *Where's your bread?*"

Everybody laughed.

"That's right," I said. "I know a woman in one of my meetings who always buys *one cookie* when she goes to the bakery. She was also embarrassed the first time—she loved those delicious pecan cookies—but they sell them by the pound. She knew that if she bought a pound, she'd eat a pound. So she got a single cookie, they weighed it, she paid her forty cents and enjoyed every guilt-free bite *more* than if she'd gorged herself on a pound!"

"Did they say anything at the bakery?" someone asked.

"When she goes in now, they take out her favorite cookie for her!" I said. "But ultimately it doesn't matter what they do. And it doesn't matter whether you're in a restaurant, out shopping, or at home. We're talking about getting people used to what they need."

A new member, a woman in her thirties with frosted blond hair wearing a tie-dyed shirt and blue jeans, actually quite slender, said: "Forget restaurants! Even at home I never knew what *a portion* was."

Knowing the Rules—And When to Bend Them

Portion control! The name of the game! Now we're talking about what could give you the power to deliver a knockout punch in that boxing match of ours! There was a time in my life when I bought smoked whitefish once a week. I insisted on having a four-ounce whitefish because I knew that from a four-ounce whitefish I'd get three ounces of fish. I made the counterman weigh the fish, one by one, until he found the exact fish I needed—one that weighed four ounces. One day I couldn't go shopping and I asked my husband to stop into the store and buy the whitefish. Of course I told him—*Four ounces. No more. No less.* As soon as he made the request, the counterman groaned and looked up at him: *"Oh, you're married to her!"* It was my way of learning, again and again, what a portion was.

"When I'm hungry," the woman in the blue jeans went on, "a potato the size of a bowling ball looks like the *one small potato* you see in the Weight Watchers® food lists. Now, I put everything right on the scale and I keep the scale out on my kitchen counter. I hope that after about a hundred years more of this, I'll automatically know what a portion is."

"I'll never be good at that," another member said. "At home I weigh it, but when I eat out, if the food is good, I eat half of whatever is on my plate."

"Yes—that's also a good rule of thumb," I agreed. "At home we can weigh and measure, but estimating what a *portion* is when we're without a scale and measuring cup gets a little tricky. The size of your palm is equal to three ounces—and I mean *your* palm, not the palm of your six-foot-three date! If you have a small palm, God is trying to tell you something—you need a smaller portion!"

"But what do you do when you're at a wedding or a dinner party and even the smallest portion of what's being served is high in calories? What do you do when there's nothing to eat?" someone asked. "When everything is in oil or covered with sauce?"

"If I'm a guest at someone's home, I don't like to make a big fuss about what I'm eating," I put in. "Let's say the salad has a very rich dressing on it or the potatoes are already buttered up. You know what? It's a one-time deal. I do the best I can and forget about it. Nobody ever got fat from having *one* salad with a rich dressing or *one* portion of potatoes with butter. It's when you eat out on a regular basis that you have to be more careful and make sure the meals work for you."

And that's the key: *How-To,* as far as I'm concerned, is *making things work for you.* FLEXIBILITY is definitely a technique: learning not to be thrown by things that don't really add up to much in the long run. A friend of mine once told me: "My son-in-law used to play chess with my daughter and beat her every time. After I got him a *HOW-TO-WIN* chess book for his birthday, *my daughter* began beating *him!*" He learned all the right moves but couldn't adapt them to the situation. So we have to see that the first principle is that these techniques are *suggestions*, not iron-clad laws. You must find your own way to apply them, you must make up your own rules—and even these you will probably have to break once in a while. Think of it as a favorite recipe that you end up changing depending on your mood or your physical condition or the time of year.

Everybody is different, and even with the very best food and exercise program, it's important to tailor it to your long-term needs. With practice, you discover exactly where you can—I was going to say *cheat a little* but make that *overeat a little.* I want to get away from that concept because we're not *cheating*, we're simply being more flexible. I've seen members who followed about ninety percent of the Weight Watchers® program and were successful. You don't always have to be one hundred percent and, in fact, it's good for you *not* to be, in the interests of survival. As one of my group members so beautifully put it: "Reality is somewhere between perfection and failure. Weight loss is not perfection. It's progress."

A woman following the Weight Watchers® program once said to me: "I've been losing weight but one thing bothers me. Plain fruit bores me and I love those bars of frozen fruit. So I've been counting them as fruit—do you think I'm right?"

"If it's working, it's right," I told her. The bottom line is that that woman was losing weight and wasn't injuring her health. By adjusting the program to meet her own needs she was assuring herself of staying with it. And in her case, what would keep her thin in the long run was that she was learning to think in terms of being on a food "budget." She was counting everything she ate, writing it down, keeping as strict a record as she would have for her checkbook. This kind of tracking is an important technique and produces great results, both short-term and long-term.

"The old me was not a fussy eater," a young man who'd lost sixty-five pounds said. "If I bought a piece of pizza and it was only so-so, I ate it anyway. What did it matter? I could always eat another piece when I passed a pizza place a few blocks away. But now that I've begun to keep track of what I eat, this slice of pizza is *it*. If I don't like what I'm eating I stop after the first bite, since a pizza is *very expensive* as far as I'm concerned: two breads, two proteins, and a fat. It *has to* be good. The crust has to be right, the sauce has to be perfect, it has to be steaming hot. I've rated every pizza store in the neighborhood with one, two, and three stars! My wife jokes that I've become like one of those restaurant critics."

The more serious we become about changing our eating patterns, the more new techniques come into play because our level of effort and inventiveness goes up. A woman in the group who'd had a very difficult life which included two years in prison is a good example of this. She'd turned other negative aspects of her life around and had decided that she could change her out-of-control eating, too.

I'd watched her go from a size sixteen to a size ten and now she had enough confidence to start dating men again. When people asked her what her secret was, she said in a very matter-of-fact voice, "I don't know, I don't really have a secret. I keep picking up new things. This month, the big surprise for me was reading labels." The drama of her self-transformation was based on techniques that seemed so simple you'd never give them a second thought. "You might say everybody reads labels," she went on, "but I finally began to read them and see what was there—and not what I wanted to be there. I stopped kidding myself. I kept remembering what you said, Rosalie—*If it tastes too good to be true, then it probably is.*"

"I've realized the same thing," said a young man who was halfway through taking off seventy pounds. "I was having these dietetic cookies every day and when I came home after the meeting last week, I asked myself: *Why do the cookies have this indentation?* So I took out a magnifying glass to read the label and discovered that the calorie value is one hundred and thirty *per serving*—and that the indentation separated what *they called* one serving from another. Each cookie was actually two servings. I was eating two hundred and sixty calories when I thought I was taking in one hundred and thirty—and sometimes, when I had two cookies, that was over five hundred calories for a light snack!"

"I could go through a pack of those in about five minutes," said a man in the group—I'll call him Fast Eater. "What they call a serving is just a joke."

"Who here couldn't?" a woman called out.

"Wait a minute—what is this, a contest to see who can eat more? Nobody's here because they don't like food," I said.

"I don't even get started eating things like that," another woman said, "because it's over in a minute and there goes a hundred and thirty calories. I think of it as a Chanel suit—sure I'd love to own one, but I just can't afford it."

"The problem is unless you really study the labels, you have no idea what you're taking in," Fast Eater added.

"Okay," I said, "so we've agreed that reading labels carefully should be somewhere near the top of any list of important techniques."

"For a long time I didn't have the patience for all this petty stuff," Fast Eater went on. A man in his early fifties, he'd dropped sixty pounds and then run out of steam for a while. Although he was no longer what you'd call obese, he still had thirty more pounds to lose but he'd stayed the same for the last six months and then made a breakthrough. "How many ounces is this, how many calories is that? I'm too busy for this kind of nonsense, I told myself—after all, I have to be out on the West Coast one week a month, and between flying back and forth and trying to keep up with the computer technology being introduced in my business, it just seemed like a stupid way to spend my time. I had more important things to do! And besides, I'm so disciplined in other areas of my life that I thought if I had to start figuring out every mouthful I eat, it would drive me crazy."

"So what changed your mind?" I asked him.

"I don't know—everything I just said was true, but then one day I heard someone say at one of the meetings: *I've been here so long that I'm a fixture.* The woman was like me: she'd lost her initial weight but she had about twenty pounds more to go. So I started taking stock. Do I want to reach goal weight or is it okay for me to be thirty pounds overweight? I had to make up my mind one way or another, because I didn't like the feeling I had about myself. I was just drifting along. It was like being in limbo."

He made the decision to take off the extra thirty pounds which meant that he had to tighten his control, so he asked me to look over the record of what he was eating. I saw at once that it would be impossible to assess things accurately because the measurements were all approximate. He'd written: A little cheese, one large health muffin, and so on. "A large health muffin" could mean anything from two hundred and fifty to twelve hundred calories. So I told him that the only way he could really know what he was doing was to start weighing and measuring things—but the idea didn't appeal to him.

"I can't stand being ruled by a measuring cup or a scale," he said. "I have to be so disciplined in every other area of my life that it's too much to start in with food."

"Weighing and measuring," I once said at a meeting. "Why do we resist it? It doesn't take more than a minute or two."

A man answered, "Because it actually tells us what we eat!"

"Yes," I said and laughed. "Last week I weighed every morsel. Our place is under construction. I said to my husband, 'It's 9:30

in the morning and I've already conferred with five men—the contractor, an electrician, a tile man, a plumber, and a painter.' And I'm so nervous, because I'm trying to figure out the colors of the rooms. Do you realize what I could have been eating during this week? So I took the precaution of measuring every bite. That was my way of dealing with the chaos."

Apart from weighing and measuring, though, I suggested that Fast Eater learn to eat more slowly, another very simple technique that leads to significant results. When you eat slowly, as opposed to wolfing down your food, you actually *experience* the meal. You focus on it. You allow yourself to enjoy the tastes and feel more satisfied with less. You can train yourself to chew longer, to take smaller bites, to put down a sandwich after every bite, to put down your knife and fork after every mouthful. You can use a demitasse spoon when you're eating dessert. When I eat, my behind must be on a chair. I don't run around talking on the phone or watch TV while eating. Remember! You're in a boxing ring! And as any prizefighter knows, concentration can win the day.

Another thing I noticed on Fast Eater's list was that he often ate the same breakfast time and again, the same dinner sometimes as often as four times a week. "It's easier that way," he said, "I don't have to think about it." But it's a proven fact that people who eat a wide variety of foods end up keeping their weight off.

Variety prevents boredom—and boredom leads to bingeing. Variety also helps you to get all the vitamins and minerals you need. In addition, it gives you greater flexibility in an environment where you yourself are not doing the cooking.

As the Boy Scouts Say: Be Prepared!

"One of the major changes for me was fresh vegetables," a young woman in the publishing business said. Her work as an editor forced her to have countless business lunches and so making these lunches "safe" was a priority for her. "Now I've eaten foods I've never tried before. Instead of glazed carrots, I've switched to broccoli rabe or roasted artichokes, which I'd never had before; I was the only one in my office who'd never tasted vegetable sushi, which I've learned to love. My colleagues are always kidding me that I should give up fiction and do a book about vegetables!"

"Didn't you know," an older woman interrupted her, "that vegetables grow in plastic bags in the grocery store?"

Everybody laughed.

"I used to think that, too! For me, vegetables were buttered corn or peas—now I admit they're starches covered with fat. I don't love everything I've tried, but I'm willing to taste anything once," the editor said, "and that's made a big difference."

Of course, this means more work. Regularly eating a variety of foods requires preparation. At one of my meetings focusing on preparation, I asked, "Tell me—what's an essential part of your day regarding food?"

A well-dressed Orthodox Jewish woman wearing a long black skirt, a silk blouse, and large gold earrings said, "You won't like this, but I do best when I'm so busy I can't think about food. And I have eleven children—so when I say busy, I *mean* busy."

Another woman, a music therapist who lives in a world of her own and dresses like a gypsy, replied to her, "I get the same way. With me, it's my music and my patients that take over. But I'm just the opposite; when I'm that busy, there's no time to think, to plan, so I tend to grab anything—and that *anything* is usually cake or chocolate. It's simple, it helps me to let off steam and feel less pressured."

A man, an ex-smoker trying to knock off forty pounds, asked the first woman: "Sooner or later, even with eleven kids, you have to eat. So what happens when you're that busy?"

"That's why I'm here!" the woman said and smiled.

"*I* do best when I know what's expected of me," I said.

"When I plan, I don't obsess about food that much," the music therapist agreed. "I'm prepared, everything is planned. I have salads that I buy by the pound. I have fish, I have fruit—it's the one part of my life where I'm one hundred percent organized."

I asked, "What can't you do without?" and a woman from the West Indies exclaimed: "Frozen vegetables!"—an answer that a surprising number of members seconded.

The mother of eleven children asked, "What about those of us who live in high volume households with lots of needs? Teenagers, a husband, and guests? I prepare my food in advance but my kids raid the fridge and so before I know it, it's gone."

"Let me tell you one thing," I said. "In my household eating my food is a federal offense. Nobody touches it. I'd brain them."

An older woman said, "When I had kids I had things just for them: whole milk, apple juice, orange juice, peanut butter, and strawberry jam—I never bring in peanut butter now—I used to eat it with a spoon."

"So your idea of preparation is *getting rid of!*" I put in. "Which is also important."

A woman dressed all in gray said, "What about a husband or boyfriend cooking a meal so we don't have to always be worrying about preparing stuff?"

"Ha!" scoffed a working mother of three who'd been quiet until then. "If I had a heart attack on the F train, my husband would still be waiting to be told what to eat two days later! It's such a big effort to cook separately for myself and for the rest of the family," she went on. "I don't have the time, it's too burdensome."

"How about one-pot meals?" someone asked. "A big pot for them and a little one for you. So you wash the extra pot—is that so terrible?"

"You can also make two versions," the woman in gray suggested. "One has the heavy stuff in it, butter or sugar and so on. If it means being thin and happy with yourself, it's worth it."

The music therapist said, "I have frozen bags of half-cup servings of rice and pasta always ready to be reheated or nuked in my freezer."

The ex-smoker asked her, "Is rice or pasta really any good when you freeze it?"

"Oh, I do the same thing," I said. "Maybe a gourmet who'd been raised eating pasta would hate it, but I'm not a gourmet and it tastes fine to me."

"Well, I *am* a gourmet and let me tell you—frozen pasta and rice is the pits! I wouldn't feed that to my husband!" a voice suddenly called out, and when I looked up I saw a long-lost member coming through the door and joining the conversation without missing a beat. I never know when I'm going to see her, because she writes the travel section for a major New York newspaper and is always flying away at a moment's notice to places like Africa and India and even Greenland. She looked fantastic—she has a great figure and knows how to dress and is an inspiring example of a woman in her fifties who is sexy, bright, and savvy.

"So what's your secret?" I asked.

"I take the time to prepare the food from scratch and you know what I've learned? I can wait! It's worth it."

"Okay, *Vive la différence!*" I said.

"My problem is that I love to cook and my new boyfriend loves my cooking. Just watching him eat can make your mouth water. I've heard that some people lose their appetite when they cook— but with me, it's just the opposite. It turns me on."

"Never underestimate the power of sensory stimulation," I said to her with a wink. "If you know you'll be surrounded by the smell and sight of delicious food, be sure you've budgeted your calories so that you can get plenty of what you want! You're a smart woman and I think you know what I'm talking about!"

I summed up the meeting by saying that preparation is the key to survival. When I first joined Weight Watchers®, I used to stick little notes to myself on the fridge—*Remember: Chew. Remember: drink water.* A good friend who was staying with me for the weekend couldn't help asking about one of them on which I'd written a cryptic message . . .

"*Rotting vegetables?*" she said with horror. She knew me very well—she knew that I'd tried *everything*, from pills to fad diets of every sort imaginable. "Don't tell me you're going to be eating *that?*"

"Of course not," I said, feeling a little insulted—although I don't know why. The idea of taking diet pills, in retrospect, is much worse than eating rotten vegetables. "I wrote it down to remember what a woman said at one of the meetings—that she can't count the number of times she had to throw out the vegetables in her fridge."

"So why doesn't she just cut down on what she buys? And what's so great about that?" my friend asked me, puzzled. She's a practical woman who runs a large jewelry business as well as being the mother of four children. She herself has never had a weight problem but for the moment she was interested in my struggle.

"Because she never *knew*. She said she kept the vegetables on hand for that *one time* it would *save her*. This woman looks fabulous, by the way," I told my friend. "To look at her you'd never know she has a weight problem. She's been on maintenance for a long time and she's gotten to the point that sometimes the idea of eating another salad or stir fry made her sick. But she said that when the feeling came over her that she wanted to eat *a lot,* then she knew that there was no way she was going to wait and go shopping. She'd turn to whatever was on hand. She knew that she had to have those vegetables in the house or else she'd end up eating whatever junk she could find."

"I see," my friend said, although from the way she said it, I know she meant the opposite.

To her that insight didn't mean much, but to me, a simple fact like that was a revelation. Up until then, when I used to go shopping "for the kids"—chocolates, cakes, candy—I never worried about overbuying. Or about price. But when it came to vegetables and fruits, it was a different story. I wouldn't *dream* of buying the red peppers I liked when their price went up to three dollars a pound that winter. But then I realized—*these are your tools*. This is your priority. How much would I be spending right now on a chocolate cake if I weren't on the program?

From Little Steps to Big Ones

Which brings me back to the important principle mentioned earlier: *Many of the steps we take to start our new life are small ones*. They're not dramatic. In the scheme of things, buying an extra head of lettuce or some pricey fruit doesn't seem to be earth-shattering. But over the long course of time, these undramatic changes have dramatic results and an amazing impact on the way we look, the way we function, who we are.

If you want *drama,* look at the before and after: a young woman who had almost ninety pounds to lose—crying all the time, ashamed to leave her house, unhealthy, lethargic; and then look at her after the weight is off—joining her husband on a hike in the mountains. You can't help being impressed. But if you retrace the steps that took her from point "A" to point "B," you'll discover that so very many of these steps seemed as unimportant as buying vegetables even though you know you may not use them.

Let me tell you something that will surprise you. When I first started being a group leader, I asked a woman in my group what she got out of the meeting that was helpful, and this is what she said: "Well, I work in the Bronx Family Court and the work and the pressure don't stop from the minute I get into the office. You can't be in eight places at the same time—but sometimes you have to be because all your cases are called at once, and it's so frustrating since each one is very important. There's a newspaper stand in the lobby of the courthouse that also sells chocolate bars and candy, so naturally I end up grabbing sweets for myself when I'm running back and forth between cases. But today the woman who sits in the back said that she looks like a bag lady every day—that when she leaves for work she loads up with bags of fruit and cooked vegetables and even sweet potatoes, for God's sake—*plus* a big lunch that she looks forward to. That was inspiring—especially coming from a woman who's lost sixty-eight pounds! I figure if she can march into a fancy realtor's office in Manhattan carrying a grocery bag filled with grapefruits and mangos, I can let my (censored) sexist boss see me nibbling on cauliflower!"

Now you have to realize that this is an African-American woman who became a lawyer despite difficult odds. She's an intelligent, determined woman who was fighting her weight problem for some time *before* she came to Weight Watchers® and joined when she saw that she was losing the battle on her own. You'd think she would have realized, on her own, that the only way to avoid that candy stand at work was to have her own foods with her! So we see, it's not only a matter of determination and it's not only a matter of intelligence, either: this woman had both.

But when it comes to food, as it's been proven with other addictions, getting support—either through the exchange of ideas at a Weight Watchers® meeting or some other support group—

is essential both to weight loss and long-term maintenance. People develop blind spots—she couldn't see something that was obvious to anyone else: if you go a long time without food and are constantly exposed to temptation, you'll give in. Period. Other people have other blind spots. This woman needed to *hear* someone in a similar situation in order to make the connections. Before I joined Weight Watchers® myself, I used to diet with short, desperate bursts of will power (followed by catastrophes). Now I have an arsenal of insights and techniques which I've learned over the years from fellow group members, from other leaders, and from *my own* group members. No one can do this completely alone.

So, let's go over the major steps we can take to get on track and stay there! Here's a CHECKLIST OF HOW-TO TECH-NIQUES that applies across the board:

1. Do you know the FOOD LISTS—the approximate value of the foods you eat? Have you learned what a portion is of each? Knowing that a potato is counted as a "bread" won't help, for example, unless you know that we're talking about a 5 oz. uncooked or 4 oz. cooked potato.

2. Do you have the right foods *already* bought and waiting in the kitchen? Remember: when you're hungry, you're not going to wait and shop for vegetables! You'll grab whatever's around.

3. The opposite of #2: Get rid of whatever foods you know will tempt you. If "they" want it, "they" can eat it outside and on their own. Don't bring in elaborate desserts for "company"—the "company" will be satisfied with fruit or something simple that won't tempt you. Don't be a martyr—be a winner!

4. Are you set up for business? That is, when you come into your kitchen starving, do you have to search for your measuring cup and food scale so that you end up just eating without bothering to weigh and measure? Is your meal ready to be heated? Are your tools—whatever they may be—ready at hand to start chopping, grating, measuring, weighing? When you're hungry, it's a danger-ous time. You should be able to fix a healthy, satisfying meal right

away. It's not the time to start shopping for food because hunger often leads you to look for a fast fix.

5. Do you eat slowly and savor every mouthful in peace and quiet? Sometimes difficult but not impossible. Do you make your eating time "special"—what I mean is NO INTERRUPTIONS! If the kids need something, if an "urgent" call comes through, have you learned to put everything on hold for the time you need to nourish and nurture yourself? I've had to accept how important food is to me. That used to be very shameful to even think to myself, but now I'm not embarrassed to say it. There's very little that I do in my mundane, everyday life that is as important to me as eating, so I better make the time for it.

6. Have you learned ways of incorporating motion and movement into your life? Notice I don't say *exercise* because when most people think of exercise they think of a long workout in the gym. I'm talking about avoiding the elevator and walking up a flight or two of stairs, parking the car a few blocks away from your destination, dancing at a party instead of hanging out by the buffet. You can make use of anything! Annoying interruptions like too many TV commercials in your favorite movie can become three- to five-minute mini-workouts. Instead of sitting on the couch munching on chocolate, you can get up and do some stretches, bends, or other simple exercises to get the blood circulating.

7. Do you know what foods you can't handle? THE MORE YOU EAT, THE MORE YOU WANT is the slogan on Cracker Jack boxes—and this is also true of certain foods which get us into trouble. I've been asked: *What is a binge food?* If I had an answer to that, they'd give me a Nobel Prize. You might be able to eat a piece of apple pie and stop there, but make that ice cream or even a certain kind of cake and we're talking about a binge. On another day you might be able to handle the ice cream—but not the apple pie. Knowing what foods set you off (and they change at different stages in your life) is very important. And again, don't lie to yourself: don't say, *I'll just have one piece* or *one taste* if you know from experience that won't happen. Any open package could be a binge food. Know your strengths *and* weaknesses.

8. Keep track. Write down everything you've eaten. This can really turn your eating patterns around. It only takes a few moments, but while it's one of the easiest techniques as well as one of the most effective, people resist it, put it off, find every excuse under the sun to avoid jotting down what they're eating. One woman who I'll call No Choice (it was either lose weight or end up *back* in the hospital) had gone through every fad diet you can imagine: the rice diet, the cabbage soup diet, the ratatouille diet, for God's sake—I'd never heard of that one before. She'd spent a fortune on doctors and pills and all kinds of far-out regimens, but she only began to make consistent and long-term progress when she picked up a pencil and paper one morning and very simply wrote down: *One egg, one piece of toast, half a grapefruit.* Now, fifty pounds and a hundred or so pencils later, she's the best example of what a simple technique can help to achieve.

9. Do you know how to maximize foods that you like but have to eat within limits? For example, a little oil can go a long way in a stir-fry. Or a portion of bread can be taken as cinnamon sugar flatbreads—they're fabulous. If I want to give myself a treat, I put a tablespoon of apricot jam on them. Or put a tablespoon of jam and a tablespoon of onion soup mix on skinless chicken before baking it—and that single tablespoon of jam will have gone a long way to making the chicken a memorable meal!

10. Learn to stop and ask yourself: *What do I need now?*—instead of heading for the food. Let me tell you something—nobody binges because they want to die of diabetes. Nobody eats out of control because they *want* to get high blood pressure or an elevated level of cholesterol or varicose veins. Nobody sits down to finish a chocolate cake with the idea in mind: *Great! So now I won't be able to fit into my clothes!* Or: *Terrific! So now I'll have three chins when they take photos at the family reunion!*

11. Keep the red light foods (foods over which we have no control) out of sight.

12. Keep platters of food off the table.

13. Serve yourself away from the table. Eat at a designated place.

14. Keep all food in the kitchen. I used to have candy dishes on the living room tables and every time I vacuumed I'd suck in a couple of candies.

15. Have someone else clean up.

You have to stop yourself and think: *WHY am I eating?* The answer often changes from one time to another and the solution often changes even when the answer is the same. One day it might be stress, and what might "do it" for you is a nap or a bath or a call to a friend. But there are no pat answers. Sure, it's easy to say: Take a walk! Go to a movie! Buy yourself something! Volunteer in a hospital! Work out with a punching bag! The point is to become attuned to your own needs and moods so that you know what you need at any given moment and don't have to turn to food. That's what thin people do.

One man in my group said that he noticed when he came home at the end of the day, he'd automatically head for the fridge. He felt tired and depleted and needed to reward himself after a hard day. But then one day he decided that he'd take a shower first and then sit down with the sports section while drinking some water or fruit juice. He'd give himself the chance to unwind without food and then start to eat in a more controlled way. He used to eat to calm down, but once he was calm—he was ready to eat again! Now he experiences his meals more fully and has dropped thirty-five pounds.

These are techniques that everybody can follow. The only requirement is that you put your mind to it. Be totally honest with yourself: if, after some soul-searching, you say, *Yes—I want to be free of this addiction!*—then you *can* do it. We can't be successful until we take responsibility, until we accept ownership of our weight issues and use our strengths to resolve those issues.

A survey asked people what their strong points were—they usually came up with anywhere from five to ten strengths. When they were asked about their weaknesses, most people mentioned more than twenty. The point is, we have strengths that we're not aware of—we use them in one area of our lives unconsciously and don't see that we have to tap them to make our weight loss work as well. It's as if we're sitting on a gold mine, but our negative self-images prevent us from making use of the gold. All we have to do is realize that we have the power, that it's there—and that success is within our reach!

CHAPTER FOUR

Curveballs

"I can resist anything except temptation."

—Oscar Wilde

There was an old Mae West movie called *Every Day's A Holiday* and those of us who have been on monthlong (or yearlong) eating binges can appreciate the irony of that title. "I'll begin to diet after the holiday," we say. But then there's the birthday party, or the illness, or the stress-producing visit of a relative . . . "I'll begin as soon as it's over!" we tell ourselves—but it's never over. It seems as if there is *always* a holiday, or crisis or irresistible temptation. We wonder if there's a conspiracy to prevent us from losing weight. But in reality, the only members of the conspiracy are ME, MYSELF, AND I—no matter what happens to us, it's *our attitude* that makes or breaks us.

Take a member of my group who had been struggling to stop her out-of-control eating for a long time. She was an assistant district attorney who gave everything to her job. She dealt with victims of child abuse, and after each case was over, she felt burned out: "I become a zombie—it doesn't matter whether I win or lose, there's only one thing I want to do—eat."

I still remember the first time she spoke up during a meeting— it was the Sunday after the Thanksgiving holiday, when many people gain back some of the weight they've lost. But this woman— I'll call her The Lawyer—was more frustrated by it than the others. She sat in the back of the room, and unlike the other women, she wore slacks and a sweater and kept shifting around impatiently in her seat, her hands twisting a scarf into a tiny ball.

"I'm listening to all of you," she said, "and it isn't making things any better. Three weeks ago, I lost eight pounds. A week later, I gained back two pounds, and the next week, I put the other six back on. I don't know if I should come here anymore. I can't get things under control, and hearing everybody talk just makes it worse. I *know* what you're going to say: you're going to tell me I should come back and that I shouldn't quit, no matter what. But sitting here and listening isn't doing me any good. I'm wasting my money because I just put on the weight."

"You *don't* know what I'm going to say," I told her, looking straight at her until she admitted that she didn't. "Anybody want to say anything?"

And then everyone began to chime in. When there was finally a pause, I said, "The real question is: what would things be like if you didn't come here? Would you be losing any weight at all? Or would your weight just be going up?"

"It would probably be going up," the woman replied.

"That's what you have to ask yourself. It could be that coming to the meetings gives you a little bit of sanity, and you might lose that if you didn't come."

Later, a middle-aged woman wearing a brown and gold silk shirt, a heavy gold medallion, and a wig said, "We're all smart ladies in this room. We could all be standing up in the front and giving advice. It's the same advice we give everybody. I used to run a high school and I would say to the boys: 'You have the chance to choose the kind of life you want. It's up to you.' I would say the same thing over and over, but do you think I ever applied it to myself? We're all smart ladies, but we're dumb when it comes to ourselves. There's a saying in Yiddish: *If people tell you you're drunk, you should go to bed.* In other words, if your friend or your husband tells you you're fat, then you're fat and that's all there is to it. There's no use walking around pretending to yourself that you're thin. We're all smart ladies, but we're not so smart when it comes to ourselves."

My lawyer member answered, "So far, I've heard one word that means something to me: *sanity*. I like that. And I like the word *drunk*. That was a good one, too." By the end of the meeting, it had become clear that what she wanted from everyone was a show of support as well as an opportunity to vent her frustration.

In any case, she *finally* managed to cut down on the post-verdict binges and everything seemed to be going well. She'd lost twenty pounds when her husband arrived with a surprise gift which threatened to destroy the progress she'd made: a two-week cruise to the West Indies. It was meant as a second honeymoon. "I was happy, Rosalie—of course I was. But at the same time, the thought flashed through my mind: *Oh well, there goes the control I've worked so hard to gain.*"

As it turned out, she had more control than she thought. When she came back, she said to me: "The food was delicious. At the end, I was very proud of myself. I'd only gained three pounds."

Reread this sentence out loud—in front of the mirror. SHE'D ONLY GAINED THREE POUNDS.

That's right—she was proud of herself. She congratulated herself. She recognized the victory—a year ago, she might have gained ten pounds on that cruise and now she had only gained three. She'd come a long way from her post-Thanksgiving depression and after the cruise, she went right back on the program and continued the slow march toward normalcy. She still had thirty pounds to lose, and she lost it.

Why? Because she didn't allow the condemning, cruel voice in her head to say, "You have thirty pounds to lose—and here you've gained three. You might as well give up. You're hopeless!" No. She said, "That's life."

When people ask me the first thing I have to do to lose weight—any amount, from five pounds to five hundred—I say: TAKE THE PRESSURE OFF.

You'll lose the weight when you lose it. Things happen and sometimes you pick up a pound or two along the way.

And we're not just talking about cruises now—we're talking about birthdays, weddings, holiday seasons, life *crises*. The point is not to make these events an *excuse* to give up hope and eat for a month or more. I've known people—and this is true of myself as well—who've eaten in anticipation of eating—that is to say, they reasoned to themselves, *I am going to eat next week anyway, so I might as well start now. Thanksgiving is just around the corner, Easter is next week, Christmas is coming—so why bother?* Of course, people can maintain or even lose weight during these times, but my lawyer friend *chose* not to. She made a choice, not an excuse, and that's what saved her.

There was a young woman who'd been in the group on and off for two years. During her first weeks at Weight Watchers®, her husband was laid off, so she had the additional pressure of taking extra work on weekends—she was involved with real estate management—as well as being the mother of two young children.

"I couldn't help it! Everything went wrong and I ate," she said to me before one meeting. I had seen her by accident near the scales. She was so ashamed and angry with herself that she'd planned on coming early, weighing herself on the particular scale she was used to, and then leaving without attending the meeting. She didn't want to see anyone. But I was early myself and it was a good thing we talked.

"My British in-laws came to visit me last week," she said. "Before I knew it, they began cooking this beautiful meal. Instead of *me* preparing it, they took over, and then that night they slept on the folding bed in the living room and I brought them their linens and towels. The next morning when I woke up, the bed was all folded away and the room was ten times tidier than it had been when they arrived. They were awake and making breakfast for the whole family, and as I was quickly getting ready in the bathroom, guilty that they had already been up for two hours and had made breakfast for everybody, I discovered that the towels I had given them were covered with rust stains. I hadn't noticed it the night before.

"So then I went down to the kitchen and they were cooking the eggs and all that was asked of me was that I toast the bagels. And for some reason all the bagels came out burned. I was really aggravated that I was burning all the bagels and I said out loud to myself: "This is a really strange morning. I don't understand what's happening." And my father-in-law said, "A strange morning?"

You have to understand that my husband's family is very uncomplaining and reserved, so that those few, simple words of mine made a bad impression. I could feel it. Which compounded my sense of being a really bad hostess.

"Anyway, my in-laws always make me incredibly nervous. They make me feel sloppy, incompetent, gross. The more considerate they are, the more nervous I get. It's almost as if I hear this voice in the background—*How could our son have chosen* her, *of all people?* The fact that they're British only makes it worse. But even if they'd been born in Brooklyn, I think they wouldn't have liked me. I'm just not their idea of what their beloved son should have as a wife.

"So what did I do? The minute I saw those rust-stained towels, I said, *Oh, my God!* and retreated to the closet with some cookies, all the while thinking, *I'll show them!*

"But what was I going to show them? My fat ass?"

Two years later. This young woman told her story to the group as an example of what *used to* bother her. She concluded by saying, "Now what do I do when expecting a visit from my in-laws? I plan extra time for a jog. I say to myself: *Get the aggression out before they show up.* I have bowls of cauliflower ready, the carrots are peeled, and the cabbage is sliced. I put my husband on notice that *he's* responsible for the brunt of entertaining his parents and seeing to their needs. Instead of eating myself into a sugar stupor, I say to him, 'Look, why don't you have something planned for your parents like a movie or a Broadway show?'

"He looks at me with that innocent expression of his—but he's not so innocent. He should have come to my rescue a long time ago—true? No. Not true, as I've learned in my long, hard struggle to lose weight. It's easy to blame him, and that way of thinking is the first step toward a relapse. *There are no victims, only volunteers,* as my sage, the wise group leader who helped me take my first steps forward, always told me. *The minute I make my fat ass his responsibility, I lose the power to change my life.*"

The trigger for this woman's eating—the curve ball—was her in-laws' visit. But of course that was only the tip of the iceberg. She had to learn a new way of dealing with her anger, a new technique, a new pattern. This kind of change takes time. We're all in a hurry, but when we slow down and realize that *the process is even more important than the result,* we're not so easily thrown off track. It didn't take a day to put on our weight, and it won't come off in a day, either—that's the attitude which paves the way for long-term success.

Changing Your Pattern

Of course, when we're dealing with family, there's always the temptation to sacrifice our needs to theirs. But we must remember our rule—*a bankrupt person cannot give anything to anyone*. One of my group members was recruited by her daughter to help out. The daughter had just given birth and wanted her mother by her side for the first weeks. But both the daughter and the husband laughed off the mother's request that there be no cake or candy in the house. I said to the mother: "Your daughter will get her figure back faster than you do if you start in bingeing. It may seem unfair, but it's food they can live without but you can't live with."

When the needs of family members become stronger, then the decisions become tougher to make; the issues are clouded with emotion. A short, delicately built woman in one of my meetings had weighed about two hundred and twelve pounds when she started. By the end, she'd gotten rid of her excess weight and was on a roll. She felt she'd turned her life around—*and she had*. Then suddenly she began eating like crazy and put back more than half the weight in a short time when she realized that her daughter was addicted to drugs.

"I just couldn't handle it," was all she said but there was so much pain in those few words that you could see the whole picture. By gaining back those pounds, she created a problem she could deal with because her daughter's addiction was something she couldn't control. There was nothing she felt she could do for her daughter. She felt helpless. So by eating she was creating a situation that she could cope with. "I know what to do when I'm over-weight," she said. "I go back to meetings, I take out the scales, I cook, I drink water, I buy healthy foods—I can fight it. But when it comes to my daughter, I'm lost."

Familiar patterns exert their appeal in many different ways. One woman left her husband of twenty years, found a small studio in the city, got a job, and lost almost eighty pounds. But she missed the intensity of her relationship with her husband, though it was self-destructive. Part of the self-destruction was the bingeing sprees they had had together. He convinced her to come back to him and she regained all her weight. Her food affected her social life, her ability to function professionally, even her health. Many times, eating partners—overweight friends or relatives—exert pressure by making us feel guilty for our success. If these people are essential to us, we have to draw the line between what will help them and what will destroy us.

Take something far less dramatic yet just as important. A man in my group needed to lose twenty-five pounds. And I mean *had to*. His weight was contributing to serious back trouble that was getting worse every year. To celebrate Easter, his mother always baked cannoli, and she was famous in the neighborhood for her cannoli. "I wanted the fucking cannoli and I wanted all of them." He was the only man in the room, and his cursing was actually a relief—we all understood those cannoli were important. They weren't *tasty* cannoli, they weren't *yummy* cannoli, they were *fucking* cannoli.

We understood how badly he wanted them. At that moment, at the holiday table, life wasn't worth living without them. So he let himself have them, and wiped out two months of weight loss in a single afternoon.

"Can you really do that?" my husband naïvely asked when I told him this story. You can tell he doesn't have a weight problem.

"Go figure it out," I said. "You lose one to two pounds a week, with a week or two of plateaus, versus thousands and thousands of custard calories washed down with liqueur—not to mention the box his mother had thoughtfully given him to take home."

So what's so good about this story? Well, the year before, he kept his Easter eating up for months. It stretched through a long, hot summer and into the fall. This time, although he had done damage—there's no denying that—he forced himself to keep coming to meetings during his bingeing and eventually he got back onto the program.

"What was the difference this time?" I asked him.

"I don't know," he said. "Maybe all this talk got to me. I had to stop kidding myself. I always used to tell myself that it didn't matter. But this time I admitted to myself that I cared." So all the work he'd done at Weight Watchers®, all the stories he'd listened to, all the talking he himself had done, had made an impression. He stopped lying to himself—and the lies we tell ourselves are the worst: *I'll binge today and walk it off later. I'll drink a gallon of water. I'll fast tomorrow* and so on and so on. He had gotten used to being honest with himself. He realized that he would have to walk to China to work off the amount of food he ate at a binge. His weekly weigh-ins had become a habit and so he forced himself to return and face the music—and that saved him.

Just as important, he didn't blame everything on Easter or on his mother's cannoli. He realized that he'd used Easter as an excuse to do what he wanted to do all along: eat. There were no cannoli at The Last Supper, nor were there chocolate-covered matzohs when Moses crossed the desert. He could have taken the edge off his appetite by eating a big bowl of salad before going to see his mother. He could have brought along a beautiful fruit platter for dessert or have asked her to make him a salad. He could have had her prepare holiday foods in a less fattening way. He could have focused on family and friends he hadn't seen for a long time. He could have done a lot of things to make the Easter holiday special without eating himself into oblivion—but he didn't. He gave in.

All right. Okay. It happens. But the fact that he picked himself up and didn't allow it to go on for months was something he could be genuinely proud of. As I always say, "When you trip and miss a step, what do you do? Catch hold of the banister or throw yourself down more steps?" He'd caught hold of the banister before it was too late.

This brings us to the second main principle of successful weight loss: DON'T JUDGE YOURSELF. Friends, relatives, co-workers think that all you have to do is stop eating; everybody knows what it means to overeat—so they have no real sympathy for this kind of problem. People make comments to help us. They think we must be dumb if we're fat, so they try to educate us by telling us about the latest miracle diet or weight loss drug, not realizing that they don't have a clue.

Obesity is a disease, but it's not a respectable disease. The same people who rush to help someone on crutches look the other way when they see an obese person. We ourselves make moral judgments: *I've been good, I've been bad*—but it's not a moral issue, it's an addiction. Only it's different from other addictions since you can't quit cold and not touch food again the way you can give up drugs.

Part of taking the internal and external pressure off is accepting yourself at whatever stage you are and seeing what you can learn about yourself right now, at this moment. RULE: *It doesn't matter what I did yesterday. The only thing that counts is what I do next.*

A courageous woman in one of my groups went to her first meeting just *before* Christmas. Usually people join afterwards when they are suffering from all the weight they've put on during the holiday, but she decided to try to get a head start. The problem was that she had sixty-five pounds to lose while her sister, who was also going to be at the family gathering, had just lost a great deal of weight.

"My sister's not saying or doing anything to make me feel bad," she said, "she just *is*. It's my problem, I know that. First my sister lost about forty pounds and kept it off for a half year. Then she joined a gym and lost another ten pounds and she looks great— she's two years older than I am, but she looks ten years younger. My husband, who's always telling me that he loves me fat or thin, God bless him, said to me—*Why do you think people are always looking? They're too interested in themselves to care how you look.* But he's naive when it comes to people—I know the truth. People will be comparing us—it's human nature."

"Look the best you can," someone in the group suggested. "Go out and buy something new to wear."

"What? Another 'fat' black suit? No, I'll find something in my closet."

"You can wear your best smile—and your best attitude," I told her. "And keep in mind that next year, if you want it, your sister's new look can also be yours."

I meant what I said—but I also knew that that gathering would be a very difficult one for this woman. I understood just how she felt. But pressuring herself about how she looked would only make her eat more.

This is true when everyday problems drive us to food, and much more so when we're beset by crisis. The amount of suffering and hardship I've seen! How can you fault anyone who says: *I can't cope since I've lost my son in a senseless accident, or I've been up nights nursing my terminally sick husband?*

In such cases I say nothing. *Eat something, you'll feel better,* is one of the biggest lies we tell ourselves. We don't feel better afterwards. The pain is still there. Each person has to come to that conclusion in his or her own time. You can't tell this to someone who's not ready to hear it. And sometimes something shocking happens to make them realize just how bad it's become: the seat belt on an airplane no longer fits; an old friend doesn't recognize them; a recent photo brings the truth home; a wedding ring doesn't fit anymore.

Or sometimes support from someone else gives us the needed push. A woman from one of my groups called me last week— she's lost eighteen pounds and has twenty to go. She's in the midst of a messy divorce. "I didn't commit suicide," she said to me. "I went underground by eating. But then what happened was that my best friend saw 'visions' of me being thin again. I'm not spiritual, but somehow when she said that to me, I became empowered."

I don't think it was the "vision" that did it. She had the power within herself all along; maybe she'd been mentally preparing herself for the change for months without knowing it. But her friend's words gave her the last push she needed.

Empowering Ourselves

Another woman told me the story of her Thanksgiving weekend. She'd been away for the holiday and allowed herself to overeat on Thanksgiving day. It was a conscious decision and not necessarily a bad one. But then she found she couldn't stop. The overeating went on for the entire weekend. The following Tuesday was the Christmas tree-lighting ceremony at Rockefeller Center where her husband worked. Now she had a choice to make: it was either go to the tree-lighting ceremony with her husband and to the party that came after, or go to her scheduled Weight Watchers® meeting.

She went to the meeting because she was afraid that if she went to the party, the overeating would continue into the New Year. The holidays had thrown her off track, but she resisted. She fought back.

Empowering yourself covers a lot of territory. A woman I'll call Resourceful told this story right after Labor Day weekend. "My niece always has the family over every year but this time I decided it would be different. I offered to bring the salad—to make sure there would be some vegetables there besides corn. But when I told my niece my plan, she tried to talk me out of it.

" 'Aunt Esther, she said to me, I want you to have a good time. I don't want you to have to work.' But she's as big as a house. And her husband, who used to be gorgeous, now needs suspenders to hold his pants up. I knew what she would serve—macaroni salad, potato salad, and cole slaw. Hamburgers. Hot dogs. You can tell what a person will serve just by looking at them."

"I know exactly what you're talking about," I said. "When I lived in New Haven I did a lot of charity work. I often attended big dinners at the end of the organization year. I could tell whether it was a thin person or a heavy person who was in charge of the menu, by the dessert. Thin women ordered sorbet with fruit. Heavy women ordered rich, gooey cake. And I should add that in those years, I always resented the sherbet—I wanted the cake!"

"The surprise was that my salad made a big hit. Everyone loved it," Resourceful went on. "It was polished off to the last leaf. It took me something like three hours to make because I bought red leaf lettuce, green leaf lettuce, mushrooms, spinach leaves, arugula, Holland peppers, good red tomatoes—everything delicious that I could think of. Plus I spent a great deal of time cutting, arranging, making it look really irresistible."

So you see, sometimes, especially when we know it's coming, we can catch the curve ball and throw it back!

When we know it's coming—but so many times, we're caught off guard. No one plans on death and illness. Last week, a woman who still has about eighty pounds to lose said this to me just before the meeting started: "Rosalie, I'm almost there!"

I perked up my ears at those words, because there was so much self-assurance in her voice that I was curious to know what she meant.

"You know I've been nursing my husband ever since we took him home from the hospital—" He'd been diagnosed with an advanced case of lymphoma. "Usually, I've stopped going to church on Sundays because I have my hands full at home. But this Sunday, my daughter came by with her husband and she said, 'Ma—come on! We're going out today. First to church and then to lunch and then to a movie. Whatever you want.'

"She'd arranged to have my other daughter stay with her father, and the two of them insisted on giving me the day off which, it turned out, I didn't realize how much I needed. I was in a very good mood when we left the house, but when we got to church and they started to sing a hymn—and it was a cheerful one, there was nothing sad about it—I began to cry. So I sat there next to my daughter and I cried and cried for the whole service and I felt so good afterwards that lunch didn't matter.

"Oh, I had a good meal out with my daughter, but what really did it for me was that cry. I know if I hadn't had it, I would have been sitting at home all day eating ice cream and cake and candy. I've heard you *say* a million times, *Get in touch with your feelings!* but until I actually experienced it, I didn't realize what it means. It felt so good to get everything out of my system that way—better than any food could have tasted. And I realize now that that's what I've been doing. Making myself into a zombie with food."

Any number of pounds she'd lost that weekend couldn't have mattered as much as that realization. She felt it in her gut and that's what would make her weight drop off during the next months. There's an old saying: *The difficulties of life are meant to make us better, not bitter.* Her husband's illness had come out of the blue. There was nothing she could do to change it. What mattered was how she faced it. It's not so much what happens to us that makes us want to eat—it's the way we react to what happens.

And we're not just talking about major problems, either, because a binge could begin from something very small—or *seemingly* small. If, the moment we feel out of control, we turn to food, it doesn't matter whether we're facing a major problem or the build-up of many small tensions and pressures. The issue is breaking the habit of using food as a coping mechanism.

Let me give you an example: A lovely woman in my group, who had been maintaining for almost a year, was thrown just by losing her car keys! She's usually on top of things—she has to be, since she's the manager of a branch of an insurance company— so you wouldn't think that such a small trifle would throw her. "I left the house and when I got to the car, I realized I'd forgotten my keys," she said at one of the meetings. "But when I went back, I couldn't find them anywhere. I had a very busy day planned. During my lunch hour, I'd promised to help my daughter, who has two young children and had to go for a doctor's appointment, so I didn't have a free moment that day. Which is no problem for me. I'm the kind of person who thrives on having too much to do. I'm very competent and usually I don't make mistakes. I was especially upset because more than business was involved. My daughter was counting on me.

"I kept feeling worse and worse as I went from room to room, and I found myself running into the kitchen every few minutes and eating while I searched for the keys. At first I just grabbed the Weight Watchers® treats I'd planned on having later that day. But as I got more nervous, I finished the whole box. And then I stopped looking and sat down and finished up a box of cereal, using half-and-half instead of low-fat milk and pouring sugar over it. Here it was, eight-thirty in the morning, and I was starting out with a whole week's worth of desserts plus my normal breakfast plus the box of cereal. And all because I'd let myself get hysterical over nothing."

"More was involved," I said to the woman—I'll call her The Manager. "It's an attitude. When something frustrates us, we've conditioned ourselves to go straight to the fridge. Big things or small things send us there. It's almost an automatic response."

"At that moment it didn't feel like there was anything else to do," she said.

"Any ideas?" I asked the group.

"I know something you could have done, not that I'm saying I would have done it," said a woman who had experienced the ups and downs of weight loss for the last five years and was now taking off forty pounds slowly but surely, half pound by half pound. "You should have relaxed for a moment and taken a deep breath!"

"I still can't deal with things like that without eating," another woman said. "Only I try to limit the damage. I turn to plain yogurt or extra bread instead of cake and ice cream."

"When I was younger," another woman in the group added, "those things made me crazy. I remember losing my checkbook and eating so much ice cream that my palate felt frozen. But I kept on eating while my husband stood there shouting at me."

"That's not usually me," The Manager said. "When the secretary wiped out a whole month's worth of records on the computer, I stayed calm. But when I lost my keys, for some reason I didn't just think to call a car service right away to go to work and to get to my daughter's. It would have cost extra money, but one way or another, I'd have to get to work—and how good it would have felt to get there without having stuffed myself! Usually, I'm calm when things go wrong."

"All right—so this time you weren't," I put in. "What are you going to do? Keep beating yourself up over it? What good will that do? I wish I had a dollar for every time I responded the way you did."

"The same thing happened to me," a woman who works for a flower store said. "I had to make a dentist's appointment and I tried to do it from work, but the secretary put me on hold and we got so busy that I had to hang up. When I called back, I got put on hold again—for a long time. I found myself reaching into a bag of doughnuts the boss keeps around and I'd finished them before I knew what was happening."

Stress! It's both a killer and one of the surest signs that you're alive! I like to define stress as an emotional or physical reaction to the wear and tear of life. Whenever the subject of stress comes up at a meeting, I ask people to tell me the purpose of a rubber band. I stretch it to show that in a relaxed state the rubber band is not doing what it's designed to do. It has be in a state of stress. But even the thickest rubber band has a breaking point, and that's when the eating comes in.

"Do you want to know what gets me hungry?" a woman said

when she heard The Manager's story. "Sitting in traffic when I'm late!"

"For me," another voice piped, "it's hearing that announcement in the subway when I'm on my way to work: *There will be a slight delay!* We all know what *slight* means. They've screwed up again."

What Does Hunger Have to Do With It?

"Okay—but it's not hunger we're talking about," I said. "We have to learn how to deal with this kind of emotional eating due to stress, boredom, happiness, excitement—because let's not forget that even positive emotions can lead to eating. Joy is a strong emotion—it can bring stress, too, because it opens you up. What we need to try to do is to break the link between strong feelings and problem eating. To learn to respond in a different way. The first line of defense is to ask yourself: *Am I Hungry?*"

"How do I know? It feels like I'm always hungry," a woman said and I sympathized with the way she felt. I've been there.

"You can start by looking at a few objective facts," I answered. "How long has it been since you've eaten? If you've eaten breakfast an hour ago you're not suffering from hunger! But if it's not that clear-cut, I have a good rule of thumb. You can tell by what you're willing to eat. If it's a salad, if anything will do, then it's hunger. If you're looking for something special then you can be sure it's in your head; it's your emotions. The first thing to do is to separate the feeling from the food. The way to do that is to scope yourself out and identify what's provoking the urge to eat."

We experience too much stress from the job, family problems, money troubles, not fitting into our clothes. From all the "shoulds". It's an inevitable part of life. Sooner or later, everyone faces it.

A grandmother said at one of the meetings, "My greatest joy is taking care of the little ones, but last week I began wondering whether it's too much for me. One of them fell against a coffee table in the house and hurt her nose and until we got her to a doctor and had the x-rays taken—thank God it wasn't broken— I was a nervous wreck. There was blood everywhere and my grand-daughter kept crying and crying. I calmed myself down afterwards with a tray of strudel I'd made for the kids—and that was the end of so much hard work at Weight Watchers®! I joined exactly one month ago when I passed a mirror in a store and saw how I looked. But now I've put everything back on in one week."

"Wait a minute!" I said. "What do you mean, *one week?* It took you a week to eat a plate of strudel?"

"I figured the diet was shot anyway," she said. "Once I'd begun . . . " And her voice trailed off.

Once she began, she meant to say, *she couldn't stop . . .*

"First of all," I said to her, "any grandmother or mother knows the kind of horror we feel when our children are suffering. It's a thousand times worse than being in pain ourselves. Of course, I could stand here and give you a lecture about getting rid of stress in a non-food way. But while there are all kinds of techniques you can use and while they do help out, I'm going to tell you something you won't read in any diet book or hear in any other Weight Watchers® meeting: *Sometimes* food is the answer. The key word here is *sometimes.* The food dulls the feelings. It calms you down. It soothes you and replenishes your energy. During a stressful time, you can count on food for all that. If you can accept that about yourself, then you'll be able to put an end to it after that one night or whatever it happens to be. Your grandchild was suffering, you were a nervous wreck, and you needed to eat.

"But if you can't accept that fact, then that plate of strudel only leads to more stress. And more eating. A whole week's worth, in fact, which is a very self-destructive act. Because when you spend a week bingeing even though you want to be thin, there's no way you can enjoy that. You're trapped, and nobody wants to be trapped."

It's a trade-off. The food gave her the comfort, and not eating it would have given her other things. More clarity, perhaps, and the ability to handle the situation more effectively; and certainly it would have given her the ability to focus on the issue at hand and to experience her feelings. I wasn't advising her to binge. *If you can soothe yourself with nurturing activities, so much the better.* I know a woman who swears by Transcendental Meditation. Sometimes non-food solutions to stress don't work. And then, the real solution comes from self-acceptance.

I'd also like to point out that sometimes delaying tactics help. Since emotional eating is usually done *impulsively*, sometimes if you can delay, even a short while, that will save you, or at least reduce the amount of food you need. Try to find an activity that will match your mood. If you are angry, maybe a brisk walk will help. If you're exhausted and nervous, take a bath, or seek comfort from someone. If you have lots of nervous energy, put on some music, dance, get on the exercise bike; *move instead of munch*. Once you begin to manage your emotions without food, it's *possible* that you can begin to look at the problem and deal with it.

If you have no one to turn to, write down all of the thoughts in your mind. I have kept a journal for years. I only write in it a couple of times a year, but it helps me to read it every so often and look back at other difficult times in my life and the strategies I used. Sometimes when you read about what was happening then, you can view the situation you're in now more objectively. It puts things in perspective. But the bottom line is that if you find yourself turning to food because of some very difficult situation, it is not the end of the world. And keeping that in mind will help you to become a long-term success.

Losing weight is a process of becoming healthy. Stress, all of our emotions, are an inevitable part of life. Misery is not inevitable, it's a choice. Love, self-acceptance, and patience are the answers. Hang in there. *No one would have crossed the ocean if they could have gotten off the ship in the storm.* I come from an immigrant background, so this saying has special meaning for me.

A story comes to mind that my husband told me. There was a child we used to see all the time in our neighborhood—a beautiful child of around eleven or so. He was really like a little angel—I'd find myself watching him playing with the other children or carrying around his little sister. He had so much grace and joy that I couldn't take my eyes off him. Anyway, over the years his family moved away and we lost track of him. Years later my husband was driving to work and he thought he saw this boy, who was then about sixteen, but he couldn't tell at first since his features were so bloated and he'd become so huge. He must have weighed about three hundred pounds. He was totally out of breath and had stopped to lean against a tree. My husband pulled over and offered him a ride. The boy slowly got into the car. It took him a good five minutes. My husband told me that when the boy said to him, "Thank you kindly," it almost broke his heart. There was so much sweetness in the voice coming from that huge, trapped mound of flesh.

My husband couldn't bring himself to say anything to the boy. What will happen to him is an open question. But whenever I hear anybody starting to talk about eating in a harsh, judgmental way, I think of that boy. Who knows what led him to such a point? But one thing is for certain—he doesn't deserved to be judged.

Since we started this chapter with the title of an old movie, let's end with one. Only let's change *Death Takes a Holiday* to *Fat Never Takes A Holiday*. We have to work *constantly* on the journey to a new life, but strangely enough our work consists of taking the pressure off, not judging ourselves, and giving ourselves room to breathe.

CHAPTER FIVE

Dearly Beloved

"A man can fall seven times. It's when he says, Someone pushed me! that he becomes a failure."
—Saying on a Weight Watchers® Calendar

"My God, have you been sick?" an overweight friend cried out in the street when she saw me for the first time after I'd lost my weight. It was a freezing cold day, but I noticed she had taken off one of her gloves and was holding a chocolate bar. "You look starved—gaunt!?"

What she didn't know was that I had waited all my life to be called *gaunt*—me, with that round face and the baby fat still on my cheeks. I was in seventh heaven, but another person might have been seriously thrown by her remarks—especially if it had been a parent or a spouse, somebody able to elicit a deep emotional response. Of course my friend was threatened by what she saw—how couldn't she be? I was able to lose weight and she wasn't. Of course it caused her pain. And the pain came out as "concern" for my health. Just to give a counterexample, let me mention that a childhood friend of mine who also saw me after that dramatic weight loss, clapped her hands and said: "Look at you! You're a sliver of a woman!", telling me how thrilled she was by my success. And I just knew from the way she said it that she meant every word.

Ah, the dearly beloved! It's a large subject that covers many different situations: sometimes it's a hostile friend, sometimes a loving relative, sometimes just a nudnik you're condemned to work with every day. Everybody knows who I'm talking about.

I've heard many stories from men and women who've struggled to lose weight that was literally killing them: *How could their friend, their spouse, their boss, their relative* NOT BE HAPPY FOR THEM? they ask with keen disappointment. They expected a hug, congratulations, a whoop of joy—and what they got was silence or a put-down.

"It made me reevaluate my entire relationship with my sister," one woman told me at a post-Thanksgiving meeting. I'll call her Nobody's Fool because of the beautiful way she handled herself. "I went to my sister's house after not seeing her since I started to diet—I was so excited that I even got there early despite the traffic. 'You look different,' was all she said to me, busying herself with hanging up our coats and setting the table.

" 'I know I look different: I lost thirty pounds,' I finally said to her. She didn't answer so I added—stupidly, I guess—'But I still have ten more pounds to lose.'

" 'Make that twenty' was all my sister said on the subject. And I began to feel terrible—until I reasoned my way out of it."

"How did you do that?" I asked her.

"Well, I *know* I look better than I did before. The simple fact that I can get up from a chair easily is proof every time I need it. I can fit into my old clothes—there's a long list of things I can do now that I couldn't do before, so I said to myself: *Screw her! I'm not going to let her destroy my self-confidence.* I realized it was my sense of being a success that was keeping me going—and she was trying to take that away from me."

There was applause in the room—so many people identified with that.

"I wish I'd thought that way fifteen pounds ago," a woman who worked for the IRS said. "I've had the same boss for the last eight years—and you know Civil Service, she'll probably stay in that job for the next ten years. For some reason, we've never gotten along. Anyway, I'd gotten down to where I was just beginning to feel good when my boss said in this really fake, so-called *friendly* voice: 'Don't go gaining it back like last time!' When I think of it now, I see that she was setting me up, trying to make me feel bad by reminding me of my past failures."

"Look, the truth is," I said, "I've learned more from my failures than from my successes—and believe me, I've had many, many so-called failures! Everybody has made mistakes, has lapses—call them what you want. Your boss could "remind" you of anything she wanted to, *but the way you think of yourself is up to you.* Nobody could make *me* see myself as a failure—and there's no reason to take in your boss's negative suggestion. Why should you play the straight man in somebody else's comedy routine?"

"What *I* would have said to her," another woman added, "is, Don't YOU go putting on the pounds I've lost."

Everybody laughed—but I questioned the wisdom of stooping to her level. "In a movie I saw on TV, I heard a line I like," I said. *Revenge is a dish best eaten cold.* As far as I'm concerned, the best "revenge" you could have had on your boss is to be thin, healthy, happy, and in control. Every time you walk through that office looking the way you want to look and feeling great, you are giving your boss the best answer you possibly could."

People like the sister of Nobody's Fool or my IRS lady's boss are threatened by change. For one thing, if they're fat (the boss was), they feel put on the spot. Sometimes they lose an eating partner. In the case of Nobody's Fool, though, the sister wasn't overweight. So maybe she liked feeling superior and relating to her sister as a fat person. Maybe there's a less dark reason—who knows and who cares? What matters isn't why *they* are bothered, what matters is that *you're* aware of what's going on. It's easier to resist these change-back messages when you can see them for what they are. Instead of eating our way into oblivion after such negative encounters, we must use our *new* knowledge to break *old* patterns.

"Whenever I see my husband's cousin, I get hungry," one woman said to me. Knowing that *in advance* gives her room to maneuver, to leave herself extra food for the occasion or just to steel herself for the encounter. Being prepared is half the battle.

Sometimes a person's basic attitude toward others changes so much that it doesn't even take a conscious effort to defend yourself. The response becomes automatic. A female police officer in one of my groups said, "Losing weight made me more assertive with my relatives." You'd think that as a police officer, that wouldn't be one of her issues, but I suppose it's one thing to stand up for yourself about weight-related issues and another thing to deal with law enforcement. "My sister-in-law gave me a box of chocolate for Christmas and I didn't thank her for it. I just turned right around and gave it to my mother. And when my sister-in-law got insulted, I told her that I didn't want it in the house. Period. She was giving me a message, so I sent her back an even stronger one."

Although one kindhearted woman in the group suggested that maybe the sister-in-law "just wasn't thinking," my answer to that was: "Well, next time, she'll think!" In my opinion, at least, the hostility here was obvious. But sometimes, ironically, the struggle is made harder by people who genuinely care about us, love us, and want to help us. That's what takes us by surprise. Not all food-pushers are "the enemy."

"I find it very hard to refuse food at social occasions," said a beautiful though very overweight woman in her forties. Since she came from a large family—three sisters and two brothers—family gatherings were important to her and food was at the center of those gatherings. "If my sister or sister-in-law has been cooking all afternoon, they're never happy if I just taste the food or even if I have a small portion. When I eat a lot, it makes them feel good. I can tell them how delicious everything is, but that has no meaning for them."

"So are you supposed to eat yourself into oblivion to make them happy?" I asked.

"It's very hard to know what to do. I don't want to ruin a birthday party or an anniversary. I feel embarrassed being the center of attention. I hate it if I seem like I'm on a diet, or if people think I'm sulking."

"Turn it around!" I said. "When people push food on you, just say: *You know, I really appreciate all the trouble you've gone to and what I've eaten is delicious. But when you keep offering me food I feel very pressured.* That shifts the responsibility onto them. You're not doing anything wrong. *They're* the ones who are pressuring *you.* If you say this in a calm, friendly tone of voice, no one will mistake it for hostility. And it doesn't even imply that you're on a diet."

A woman who works for an important political figure showed up in my Manhattan meeting one day with an interesting comment about "food pushing." She lost between ten and fifteen pounds several years ago and is constantly struggling to keep them off. I always say that the number of pounds a person has to lose doesn't really indicate how difficult a weight problem they have. Nobody knows how hard those people have to work to take off that weight, be it five pounds or fifty. If you eat two cookies and can't stop, you have a weight problem—period.

I always know this woman's frame of mind—I'll call her The Advance Lady—by the way she's dressed. If her blouse is tucked in or if she's wearing something belted, I know she's in control. Otherwise, she's been bingeing. On the day in question, she was definitely in control.

"Over the weekend I flew to St. Louis to see my mother," she said. "It was her birthday. Although I looked forward to the trip, I dreaded the effect it would have on my eating. My mother is always telling me to try this or taste that, always making a big point of how worn out I look and how I should take better care of myself. And in her book, taking better care of myself means eating.

"Anyway, the weekend went the way I expected it to. I didn't argue with my mother—after all, it was her birthday—but her comments and attitude made me tense all the same. Finally, just as I was about to leave, she handed me a package of sandwiches she'd made up for me to take on the plane. Thick slices of buttered bread with cheese. And homemade muffins that I'd been resisting all weekend. Just before I left, she handed me the bag and said, 'Here. For later. Just in case you get hungry'—a phrase I must have heard a million times in my life.

"And all of a sudden, something clicked: *So what if I'm hungry?* I've been a lot worse things in my life than hungry. I've been broke. I've been jilted. I've been sick. If I've lived through all that, I can live through being hungry. All the way home, I thought through this *dread* of hunger, and I think I worked something out."

"And I bet that the next time you see your mother, her words won't have the same effect on you," I said to her. "People can only get to you when you're vulnerable." The Advance Lady, for all her sophistication, still had to come to terms with childhood patterns, and on that weekend trip, she'd taken a big step forward.

Nudnicks, Nudges and Nuisances

All right! So much for the "food pushers"! The opposite types—I call them "the jailers"—are just as big a headache, though in a different way.

A woman who had reached goal weight and who wanted to help her daughter, who was also overweight, kept nagging at her to "go easy", to try some salad, to go for a walk, etc. "One day my daughter turned and glared at me," she said to me after a meeting, "and then shouted: 'Leave me alone! Anything you say just makes it worse!' And so I never said anything after that. I wanted to cut off her hand below the wrist, but I never said a word. Do you know how painful it is for me to be thinner than my daughter, to see her gaining weight every week—and to have to be silent?"

Yes, it's painful, but she's made the right decision. Sometimes you just have to back off and hope for the best.

A man from Australia in one of my groups was told by his doctor that unless he lost fifty pounds, he was heading for a second massive heart attack—he'd survived his first some years before. A routine checkup revealed that he weighed three hundred and fifty pounds. Before that, he'd always weighed in at three hundred—he thought he was "holding the line," but that visit to the doctor made him investigate and he discovered that his scale simply did not go higher than three hundred. He'd been kidding himself.

"We were going to visit my wife's brother and my wife put the word out—she let them know that this time I was *serious*." So when dessert time came around and everyone was given a piece of apple pie, the man—I'll call him my Aussie—was handed a plate with some fruit on it, along with some "dietetic goo" that his sister-in-law called "pudding."

"It was insulting and infuriating, Rosalie," he said. "During the war, I was in charge of an entire company—but suddenly it was as if I were a baby and couldn't be trusted to take care of myself. My sister-in-law bakes terrific pies, and I'd purposely left myself enough calories to take that into account. But when I asked for a slice, she said in a patronizing way: 'Should you really be having that?'—Thinking, I guess, that she was helping me."

"What did you do?" a member asked.

"I know I should have explained to her what I was doing—" he started to say.

"No," I disagreed, "you don't owe any explanations to anyone."

"Anyway, I won't repeat what I said, but it started a big fight. Plus, afterwards I had an ice cream soda to calm down—and *that* I really shouldn't have had."

"All right," I said, "it's over. The fact of the matter is you're sitting right here. You've come to the meeting and that's a sign that you're back on track. Don't worry about yesterday, think about tomorrow."

What did my Aussie's relatives expect, that he would go without any dessert or treats for the year or two it would take him to lose the weight? The healthiest and most nutritious eating plan has to make room for an occasional indulgence. His asking for that apple pie was a sign of health: *of course* he could fit a piece of pie into his eating program; that pie was a way of keeping him satisfied and stopping him from bingeing. What he'd done as an overweight person was very hard: he was eating pie in public *the way a thin person does*. He knew how much weight he needed to lose—and he was very aware of the fact that his relatives knew how much weight he had to lose. He knew they might be thinking: *How can he eat that, looking the way he looks?*—or worse. But he was committed to a new pattern. He deserved pleasure, he'd decided, so he figured out how many calories the pie was, he cut back elsewhere, and then the "experts" made him feel bad. Their intentions might have been the best in the world, but what matters is the effect their words had on him.

So what could he have done—what do *you* do in such a situation? Part of being prepared is thinking through these issues in advance, having a plan, knowing how you're going to respond. If it's a first-time offense, you might simply say, politely but firmly:

"What I eat is my business. Let's not talk about it." If those people are really trying to help, it won't happen again. If it does, you may have to lay down the law or give up eating with that particular person.

I like to give people a formula to help them stand up for themselves in this kind of a situation without hurting others. I advise them to think of using sentences that have these words in them: *When you . . . I feel . . . because . . .* So in our Aussie's situation, what I would have said was: *When you ask me* Should you really be having that?, *I feel angry because* I *want to be in control of what I eat and what I don't eat.* I *want to make the decision.*

One man, who'd lost forty pounds with the program and was on his way to reaching his goal, said: "Whenever I saw my brother, he would always ask why I couldn't lose the weight on my own. He had also been overweight, but he said all he'd had to do was to cut his portions in half. I'd tried that myself, but it hadn't worked for me.

"Whenever he came over to visit, he would throw up the fact to me that more women than men joined Weight Watchers® and then add for good measure: *I'm not a joiner!* In the beginning, it bothered me until finally one day I just said to him: "Well, I *am* a joiner—so big deal!" and laughed at him. I had to realize that he and I are not the same people and how he loses weight has nothing to do with me. And do you know what? I think since he sees he can't get to me, he's stopped needling me."

Some people wouldn't have been as patient as this man was. I know that I, for one, would have shut his brother up right away. But however you choose to handle this kind of situation, *don't* suffer in silence. Self-respect is a crucial part of this process: I'd rather open my mouth and upset other people than keep it shut and upset myself. That's part of learning TO PUT YOURSELF FIRST, a subject I'll go into later on. The truth is that your weight loss will often lead to a difference in the way you relate to other people and that difference often leads to tension until they accept the new you.

Dealing With the Big Picture

If these people happen to be your mother or your mother-in-law, your father or your spouse, then you're looking at a long-term problem: you have to look at the whole pattern of the relationship. You have to see their interference in terms of what's *really* going on between you and deal with the big picture.

For example, sometimes weight is a hook people have into you. There was a woman whose husband was after her to lose weight—he used to bring it up all the time, when they were alone, when they were in public. It wasn't just "Are you allowed to have that piece of cake?" it was "You should know how good she used to look when she was thin. She was a real knockout."

Finally, she decided to take action. She had two small children at home, plus she was paid to take care of the neighbor's children. It wasn't exactly day care, but she always had three or four small children on her hands. The only way she could get to her Wednesday night meeting would be for her husband to cover for her when he came home, but on Wednesday nights—for some strange reason, right?—he always showed up late, making her miss the meeting. What she finally came to see was that he enjoyed putting her down. He said he wanted her to lose the weight, but he didn't. The weight change shook up their whole relationship. It made her seem more powerful, more beautiful, more in control.

It began with her demanding that he be home on time Wednesday nights, and it ended up with her seeing that she needed more free time for herself—time just to get out. She also began to feel good enough about herself to stop her husband in his tracks if he tried to put her down, whether they were alone or in public.

"Looking back on it now," she said, "I think I have a better marriage. We'd fallen into a rut that wasn't good for either of us."

Sometimes, though, we get angry with those around us and make *our* problems *their* fault: as a general rule, when nobody around you measures up, it's time to check your yardstick, as the old saying goes. That's one side of the coin, but the other side is that mothers, husbands, In-laws & Co., often send all kinds of subtle and not-so-subtle Change-back-to-the-way-you-were messages. It might be: *You were so much more fun before you went on the diet*. It might just be that they ignore how good you look after losing all that weight. It might be to bring you all kinds of tempting foods and to insist you try *just one bite*. They aren't always out to sabotage us; sometimes they want us to reach our goals and just don't know how to be helpful *in the right way*.

But sometimes they do. A woman I really root for—she's come through so much in her life, having been widowed twice, the first time at a very early age—lost about eighty pounds in a year and a half (she still has forty more to go). The way she rewarded herself was that every Sunday, after weighing in, her boyfriend would take her out to a nearby restaurant in Queens—one week sushi, one week Thai food.

"I feel very guilty about something, Rosalie," she confessed after the meeting (people often do that even though I don't wear a Roman collar). "My boyfriend spent over seventy dollars on me last Sunday."

"Good for him! What was the occasion?"

"That's just it. There was no reason for him to be so extravagant, but he insisted. You know, last week I had been really good and was looking forward to my sushi lunch. But when we got to the place we usually go, it was closed for repairs—a water main had broken nearby. We'd had a hard time finding a place to park, but anyway we got back into the car and drove to another place someone recommended about a half hour away. But when we got there, we found out that the sushi chef hadn't shown up yet—so no sushi. As it turned out, there was a third place not so far away but it just wasn't our day—that restaurant didn't open till five. I'll tell you, Rosalie, I was ready to give up—I figured I'd have something else, why make such a big production of it? Why not just forget it?"

But her boyfriend wanted to show her how much he supported her weight loss efforts—really, how much he honored her. They were due at his parents' house to go over some legal papers, but he insisted they get back into the car. They finally found another restaurant, but a very fancy one.

"I would have been happy with my regular place—but let me

tell you, I never had such good sushi. I loved every mouthful, and it really made me see how much my boyfriend cared."

It wasn't just that her boyfriend cared, though—I have seen many boyfriends or husbands caring and not doing what he did—it was that he cared *and* he understood. There are many times when other people do love us and do care about us, but just can't really understand what we go through.

I'm reminded of one of my mid-winter meetings—during a snowstorm (when, by the way, only the very dedicated turn up). A woman I'll call my Ad Lady brought up a situation that was making her miserable. She was in charge of very important campaigns for a major New York advertising company.

"I'm used to dealing with pressure, deadlines, the works," she told us. "I can handle any situation, so why can't I handle this one? I go to my aunt's house to visit when I have time. She's really a great old lady and I love seeing her. Whenever she hears I'm coming, she spends hours making this delicious strudel with tons of apples, nuts, butter, and sugar. If I should try to suggest using a butter substitute or Sweet and Low instead of sugar, she says emphatically: *It won't be strudel anymore.* Since I was a kid the strudel is her way of telling me she loves me. What am I supposed to do? Give up visiting her?"

There was silence in the room for a moment. A lady—I'll call her Doing Fine since she has been on maintenance, with ups and downs, for the last eight years—said thoughtfully: "Well, if it stops with a piece of strudel or two it won't kill you. You can even lose weight that way—I know I have. But if you use that one piece as an excuse to binge for a week, then you know something else is going on."

"That's just not true," The Ad Lady said resentfully.

"Wait a minute," I said, "you mean that's not true *for you*. Everybody has their own experience."

"Well, with me, that's how I am," she added. "Once I go off track with a piece of strudel, I can't get back on. I just eat and eat and eat. Sometimes I even end up bringing cake and ice cream with me to work and eating in my office."

"I wouldn't call eating a piece of strudel *going off track*. That's your first mistake. You've got to make allowances for all kinds of treats to survive in the long run." These words came from a middle-aged, overweight woman who has had many "campaigns"—I'll call her The Old Trooper."

"But I'm not that way. With me, it's all or nothing," The Ad Lady said.

"Listen, if you're going to be that way, forget it," The Old Trooper answered. "Food's not heroin or crack. You're going to be eating for the rest of your life. Are you telling me that you plan on eating only lettuce for the next forty years?"

Everybody laughed, even The Ad Lady.

Doing Fine added: "I'll bet you anything that if your aunt gave up baking strudel, it would be your sister's lasagna that would set you off instead."

"No, no, no," The Ad Lady said, "it's the strudel that kills me every time. I'd be on track if it weren't for that."

A woman who had been silent at all the meetings so far—a short, attractive black woman who runs a clothing store—said in a quiet, thoughtful voice: "There must be a way to tell somebody you love and who loves you that the strudel is not good for you."

"I can't think of how to say it," The Ad Lady answered impatiently.

"I used to have that with my relatives all the time," a very overweight young woman in her twenties said. "The I-made-this-just-for-you routine. But when I stopped eating it, they stopped making it. It was as simple as that."

"She's an eighty-year-old woman!" The Ad Lady countered. "Of course I could get her to stop making it. But I know what it would do to her inside. You should see how proud she is of her strudel."

"What's more important to you—her feelings or your weight?" the overweight young lady asked.

"They're *both* important to me," The Ad Lady said.

"Okay," I said. "Your aunt's not going to change. There's no way you're going to get a plate of carrots and celery next time you visit. It's like the old song, "Something's Got to Give." You have to think about what it is in the situation that set you off."

"I guess it's the one place where I can really let myself go," she said in a lower voice. "I like the way my aunt takes care of me. I love my job but I'm always involved with one crisis or another there. There are many nights where I don't get home until eleven or twelve o'clock."

"My guess is that you have to find more times to let some of that tension go," I said. "More ways, I mean. Your aunt's house shouldn't be the only place you feel taken care of."

The woman went through a whole series of changes that year. Ironically, some of the choices she made produced even more stress. The aerobics class she took (and then dropped), for instance, made her even more nervous because she was competitive and driven and had to be the best. When she started jogging she had the marathon in mind. Her aunt was only part of the problem; the other part was her own perfectionist nature. When it comes to food, the people who succeed over a long period of time are the ones who give themselves leeway, who let themselves savor the occasional strudel or pie or whatever it happens to be. So dealing with her aunt meant dealing with herself.

Other People Don't Change

RULE: OTHER PEOPLE DON'T CHANGE; THE WAY WE REACT TO THEM HAS TO CHANGE. In the case of The Ad Lady, she's maintaining. She hasn't reached her goal weight yet, but she hasn't put back the initial twenty pounds she lost, either. One big achievement is that she now has insight into her problem. Maybe one day she will learn to give to herself more, to nourish herself better so that when she visits her aunt she won't feel so deprived.

Here we're dealing with the case of a relative who just doesn't understand. But many times we have relatives or spouses who do understand—*but who just can't be there for us emotionally.* For example, a woman in my group, in her thirties, told me a story that took place when she was in college. "I was a freshman, I was away from home for the first time, and although I wasn't so far away—about two hours north of the city—I felt very unhappy and turned to food. It wasn't that I couldn't do the work, I was always on the dean's list. But I guess I was socially backward. I was shy, I hadn't even been allowed to go on dates before, and now I was thrown into a world where the kids were much more sophisticated than I was. My eating only made things worse. I'd always been a little overweight, but this pushed me into a different realm completely: I put on twenty pounds in the first two months. And then one day in November, my grandfather died—he hadn't even been sick—and I was called home to the funeral. You know, Jewish funerals always take place right away. I was called at ten in the morning and told to be at the funeral that afternoon at two.

"I ransacked my closet looking for something to wear and I finally came up with God knows what—an old black sweater that really didn't fit right and a shapeless Navy blue skirt that didn't close—I thought the sweater would hide that. I knew I looked bad, but it was when I arrived home that it hit me full force. My mother looked at me and there was *such* disappointment in her eyes that I will never forget it. She didn't say a word but I knew she was thinking, *Is this how you come to your grandfather's funeral?*"

Of course, in the best of all possible worlds, the mother would have thought of her daughter's situation, how much pain she had to be in to have gained all that weight. But at that moment, she was going through her own feelings and what a saint she would have had to be to react that way. Her own parent had died, the family was gathering, and she felt humiliated at the way her daughter looked. And that's what happens sometimes even with people who love us: they have their own troubles and they can't give us the kind of support we need. We have to remember that: if help comes from outside, that's great, but we can't always expect it. We have to learn to find the strength within ourselves.

"I started overeating when I was just a kid," said a young woman who works for one of Manhattan's most prominent art dealers. She was well groomed and very well dressed though she carried an extra forty pounds. "When I was a teenager I used to wake up and find pictures of thin models next to my pillow—my mother and father never let me alone on the subject. When we went shopping they always took me to see what the *other* kids would be able to buy before we went to the Chubette Department. Whenever I tried to lose weight, something in me would rebel—

the amount of pressure they put on me made it impossible for me to lose a pound. It took years before I was able to decide to lose weight *for me*, not for them. Even now when I visit my mother— my father passed on—she looks me over critically although she doesn't say anything."

"I hear you," a young woman in her thirties said. "I had the same kind of situation, only it started a little later. When I was a kid I didn't have weight problems. Our high school—I was raised in LA—had these beauty pageants and my father used to make me enter them—"

"They still have them," a woman from North Carolina said. "My niece was in one last spring."

"There's a good side and a bad side to them," the young woman went on, "only I think that when the parents start pushing their kids, it causes a problem. Both my parents, but my father especially, were totally into it. In the beginning I was runner-up in a few and I even won once, but I think all the talk about how I looked finally started me bingeing. It was a way out of it—nobody wants someone else breathing down their neck. The trouble is that now I have to learn to care how I look for myself, not for some panel of judges."

"I had just the opposite kind of pressure from my mother. She was always pushing food on me," another member, a very angry woman in her forties, said. "I broke down and ruined a whole month's work because of her," she said at one meeting. "It's her fault, it's the way she raised me. When I was upset about anything she would always say *Eat something and you'll feel better*. When I visit her or just when we talk on the phone she has a terrible effect on me. She just sets me off."

Now, I normally don't like to intervene in other people's lives, but I said to her, "There's a statute of limitations! You've been out of your mother's house for thirty years now. When are you going to take responsibility for yourself?"

A young man in the group put in: "That may be true, but if you clip a bird's wings early, it'll never fly."

"Yes, but it can still hop from branch to branch," an older lady answered him. "There are all kinds of adjustments a person can make. You can be given a problem when you're young, but it's how you deal with it that matters."

One woman spoke up: "I couldn't agree with that more! I'm a widow, a grandma many times over, and I still have food issues with my mother. She's *still* telling me what to do and it *still* gets to me. The other day I told her I wasn't coming over because I didn't want to give her my cold and she told me that if I ate better I wouldn't be getting sick so often. Do you think I didn't eat more than I usually do after that? Of course I did—out of aggravation! And maybe it was my way of listening to my mother, too. Only instead of a box of chocolates, what I ate was an extra portion of fish and a baked potato with low fat sour cream on it."

The angry lady shrugged this off. "Yeah," she went on, "but you have to know my mother—" I saw that she wasn't yet ready to consider any alternative to the way she was looking at her situation.

Of course it would be wonderful if her mother was helpful or even just backed off and let her handle her weight problem on her own. Of course it would be wonderful if every boyfriend or husband (or wife) was as helpful as the one who went from sushi restaurant to sushi restaurant to reward his partner. When I told that story to one of my members, she shook her head and said, "Whenever I bring up my weight to my husband all he says is, 'Shut up! I've been listening to you talk about your weight for thirty years!'" Of course, an appreciative and supportive husband would have made her struggle easier. But the bottom line is, she was able to do it herself. That's what we have to remember.

It's often when we stop seeking approval that we get it. But whether or not we do, we have to remember what Will Rogers put so beautifully: *If you depend on applause, you're putting your happiness in the hands of other people.* It's time for us to take our destiny back into our own hands.

CHAPTER SIX

The Binge—From Tragedy to Triumph!

The second day of a diet is much easier than the first. By the second day, you're off it.

—Jackie Gleason, comedian

"For years I never got dressed," a member said. "No, I'm not a nudist, and I haven't lived in a Turkish harem, thank you very much—I'm a happily married woman. I mean that I shlumped around in muumuus and dusters. Putting on a slip felt like wearing a tourniquet, so you can imagine the kind of clothes I bought." I call this the "Japanese Fish Phase" because it reminds me of a Japanese fish I read about in some magazine: if you put it in a small bowl, it remains small. Give it a huge tank, and it'll grow to ten feet. The sky's the limit—that's the way it is with these loose fitting, flowing sacks. There's endless give, so we never have to remember what's happening to our bodies. My member went on: "If I had to run out to get something at the supermarket, I'd throw a coat over my muumuu—in the middle of winter yet— and put on some galoshes."

"And you were ready to NOT face the world," I said. Because that's what we're doing when we act this way: we give up on appearance, and part of that surrender is trying to forget that we have a body at all.

So we're talking about getting undressed to binge—a warning sign, like thunder on a humid summer's day. When you dress like a fat person, it's so much easier to eat like a fat person. This is one advantage that someone in the business world has over a housewife or retiree—they are forced to conform to a dress code. As they gain weight, every morning they have to confront a closet full of clothes that don't fit. But while clothes can help bring the truth home, they never stopped anyone determined to binge. There are many people who feel pressured at work and who turn to food as a way to keep themselves going—they grab a piece of cake as a deadline approaches or they give in to the Danish and coffee being wheeled from office to office.

Mothers and housewives who stay at home say: *If only I had a regular job to go to! There's no way I'd be bingeing. It would give me the structure I need. I would be away from the fridge. I'd be forced to get out and get dressed.*

People at work say: *If only I could stay home! I'd have time to prepare healthy foods for myself, to eat what I wanted, when I wanted. I'd be able to exercise more, to go for walks. I could really take care of myself.*

But the truth is, they're both right—and they're both wrong. If food has become the answer for a person, a way of dealing with stress, change, a way of handling emotions—a coping mechanism—then what's the difference if they're at work or at home?

And emotions are usually the trigger for a binge because—
RULE: THE MIND EATS BEFORE THE STOMACH DOES!

Of course a person is in more danger of bingeing when they're ravenous—when they've gone too long without eating, it's easier to lose control. But this is because their physical hunger has stirred up the *feeling, the emotion* of being deprived. When they let themselves go through a stressful or busy day without eating, the binge afterwards isn't the result of hunger—a bowl of steaming vegetable soup, some chicken, steamed vegetables, some fruit takes care of hunger—it's because they need to *feel* nourished, they need to release all the pressure they've been under. That day's deprivation stirs up other feelings of deprivation—then they turn to ice cream and cake to make up for those feelings. The bottom line is, if what you're feeling can't be satisfied with a healthy meal then hunger isn't what's gnawing at you.

Let's start by defining a binge. What makes it different from an occasional overindulgence? Although there's no one single form it takes, usually it's a large amount of food eaten very quickly, way beyond the point of comfort—alone, out of control, and usually followed by feelings of hopelessness, humiliation, and despair.

Even if bingers start out in a good frame of mind, by the end they are usually in a stupor; they feel bloated, in the power of food, and are often in another world. One woman traveling abroad on vacation told me that she once ate so much pizza that she ruptured something and had to be taken to the hospital. Another woman went into such a deep sleep that her husband thought she'd passed out. It's a serious matter which can have dire physical as well as emotional consequences ranging from heart disease to diabetes.

I've often asked at the meetings: *How do you feel just before a binge?*

These are some of the answers I've gotten to this sixty-four thousand dollar question:

Nervous.
Tired.
Stressed out.
Put upon.
Bored.
Overwhelmed.
Very, very fat.
Hopeless.
Needy.
Bargaining with myself.
Happy.
Excited that I'm going to eat what I want.
Criminal pleasure.
I got a promotion—food was the icing on the cake.
My father-in-law died; I needed to eat until the funeral was over.
I had my first grandchild—I ate during my daughter's labor, I was so nervous! And then I ate for a week after the christening—I was so happy!
The warm weather began—and somehow it unsettled me. Whenever the season changes, it doesn't matter from winter to summer or summer to winter, I find myself eating more.

"You want to know how I feel just before I binge?" asked a

large man in his fifties who became serious about weight loss after a massive heart attack. "I'm on the prowl. Sometimes it's in the middle of the night and I get up out of bed and go down and look through the kitchen shelves and open the door of the fridge and just stand there. I can't sleep. I'm not really hungry, but I'm not satisfied, either. I don't plan on gaining five pounds—I feel like having *something*. I never say, *I'm going to overeat now*. I never think of it as a binge."

"What do you think of it as—a workout?" the group "toughie" asked.

A young woman in the group came to his defense: "No, I know what he's saying—I'm exactly the same way. I just want *something*. When I feel like that, it means trouble. I eat whatever—the ice cream, the cake, the cookies—and it doesn't do the trick. So I think: *maybe something salty*. That doesn't hit the spot, so I go back to the chocolate cookies—but somehow that wasn't what I really wanted. I don't know what's wrong with me, I don't know what I really wanted, what spot the food is supposed to hit, what trick it's supposed to do. *What do I really want?*

Each and every one of the answers on our list—*tired, nervous, bored, excited, stressed out, anticipating*—could end with this cry: *What do I really want?* because people turn to food when they are at a loss. We can't deal with stress—and even happy events are stressful—so we eat. We can't face the pain of a loss, or the pressures of a job, a decision that is tearing us apart—so we eat. We can't say NO to demanding friends or relatives—so we eat. Of course, when the binge is over, we still have to face whatever it is we're running away from, and not only that, but face it with extra weight and the job of getting back into control. At the moment, though, we can't think of that. We all have selective memory: we don't want to remember how we feel when the party is over. All we experience is *wanting something* and we are not used to fighting off that impulse. But we *can* fight it off, and the more we resist it, the better we become over the years. Success breeds success—while just the *feeling* of failure *leads to* failure.

Take the case of a woman I'll call The Swimmer, since she was on the swim team in school and remained a fan of swimming. During a recent meeting that focused on bingeing, she said: "I binged all March. I didn't exercise, didn't get out of bed except to go to work. And then I thought: *I'm thirty-six. I want to enjoy the summer. I want to go swimming and lie out in the sun. This year I want to be able to wear a bathing suit and not die of shame—Memorial Day is only six weeks away.* So I got back on the program—and the first time I weighed in, it turned out that I had only gained three pounds even though I'd been eating like a pig."

"Three pounds?" I said. "You couldn't have been eating like a pig. If you told me that you had gained five pounds in four days, I would believe you. What exactly did you eat?"

"A lot of fruit. I ate oranges—up to eight a day. Bowls of cherries and grapes. And I had yogurt with them."

"Look at that!" I said. "Think how you've changed! What used to be *a little snack* is now a *binge*—enough to put you to bed. You see? We *do* change."

"But it's hard to *feel* the change," she answered. "I still keep all my 'fat' clothes and my 'middle-size' wardrobe. I'm afraid I might start bingeing again and need them."

"Throw away the 'fat' clothes!" two or three members called out.

"That's what everybody tells me, but I can't bring myself to do it. Last week I put them in storage."

Until The Swimmer returned to the meeting, she thought she was a failure even though, in fact, hers was a success story. After all, the damage she'd done in her month away was minimal—she'd gained only three pounds *plus* she'd kept off the other thirty! The fact that summer was coming, the memory of other summers when she was fat, renewed her resolve. But many people I've seen, in her position, turn to nonstop bingeing because they think "all is lost"—though in reality they might not have gained even as much as The Swimmer's three pounds!

They were locked into the old all-or-nothing mentality which frequently takes over after a binge, even if it's only a small one. And then their feelings of failure make them continue to eat until they've drifted back into their old habits, one by one. The way they see themselves becomes a self-fulfilling prophecy and gradually they put back all the weight they've lost.

Gaining—Perspective

We have to learn that a binge is not the end of the world. We're talking about perspective. We're talking about the right attitude. Say we eat more than we normally do—maybe it's a binge, maybe it's just a bingette—either way, the first step is to accept what we've done: *All right! So I've had a plate of French fries! I've had a milkshake. Okay! So I've eaten yogurt and fruit nonstop for a month!* It's over and done with. By looking back, we turn into a pillar of salt as surely as Lot's wife. Dwelling on our lapse is nothing but self-sabotage. The solution is to return to the meeting, pick up a measuring cup, put on our walking shoes, and begin again. The alternative is misery—more of the same. We know where we've been. We don't want to return there. And if we just think of that, we will realize that *we must go forward.*

"It's hard to change yourself," a woman who'd lost about half her extra pounds said after hearing The Swimmer's story. "You get used to being heavy and when the pounds start coming off, you get nervous and start to binge. It's almost like a friend, especially since I've retired. I'm having a difficult time making the adjustment and when I get depressed, the only thing I want to do is eat. It's hard to give it up."

But it's not so hard once we've developed other "friends"—by which I mean people, activities, or even other foods that we can turn to when we "just need something." Going to a movie or a play, calling up someone you like but have been out of touch with, cooking up a delicious dessert that fits into your eating program takes more effort than reaching for a piece of cake, but the effort pays off.

An actor who made a living in the New York theater and invited me to one of his performances told the group that in the past he had lost over one hundred pounds and immediately felt the need to put back fifteen because he missed his insulation, his padding, the layer between him and the world. Another group member said that during the times in her life when she felt most vulnerable— during a divorce and after the death of her mother—she noticed that putting on weight gave her a sense of security. It was as if she'd wrapped herself in a thick blanket.

But we're not just talking about the emotional crisis which sends us to food—we're talking about changing the way we deal with the simplest physical discomforts. *I am tired, I am cold, I am thirsty, my clothes are too tight, my feet hurt*—all of these often are translated to the brain as: *I want to eat. If someone is tired, why don't they just go to sleep?* you might ask. Because a person who has been resorting to food for a long time, a person who thinks of chocolate or cake as a cure-all, has to learn to stop and ask: *How do I really feel now? What do I really need now?* Distinguishing between being *tired* and wanting to eat, between being *thirsty* and going for that gallon of ice cream, is a first step. And because it's such a basic step, many people overlook it and stumble into bingeing without realizing that a nap or a foot massage or just getting off their feet for an hour is what they really need at that point.

One woman, I'll call her The Young Mother, found herself with three young children (two of them twins) a short time after she got married. She coped as best she could, but she'd never really thought through her choices. She basically fell into a certain style of life that included eating sweets and chocolates and cakes when she felt deprived until at the age of twenty-nine she was sixty pounds overweight.

"I was raised according to the Protestant work ethic as it applies to immigrant parents," she said at one of the meetings. "Just the other day when I went home, my mother was telling me about her tenant upstairs—my mother disapproves of her because she goes to sleep every afternoon when her two-year-old takes a nap. The idea of going to sleep in the middle of the afternoon when you're not sick—just taking a nap because you're tired—would never cross my mother's mind. You keep going, that's it—and, of course, there's nothing wrong with grabbing cake and candy if you need some energy. That's what it's for. For a long time, that's the way I functioned, too, until finally I was just so sick of being fat! I couldn't stand the way I moved around anymore, I couldn't stand the sight of myself in the mirror. So one day, just as I was about to binge, I took your advice: I stopped for a second and asked if there was anything I could do for myself before I ate. I didn't think of it as *instead of* eating but *before* I ate. It was—what did you call it again, Rosalie?"

"I call it the window of opportunity," I put in. "There's usually a very short time, a few seconds right before the binge starts, when you have a chance to talk yourself out of it. To pull yourself back."

"Well, that's exactly what I did this time. I kept asking myself, *What do I want?*"

"And what was the answer?"

"Two weeks in Hawaii!" she said and everyone laughed.

"With or without your husband?" someone called out and there was more laughter.

What this young woman ended up doing, though, was better than two weeks in Hawaii: up until then, she'd only hired a baby-sitter when there was what she called a "real" reason for it. When her mother was sick and she had to help take care of her, or when someone gave her a big sewing job (she made money that way part-time), then and only then would she pay a local high school girl six dollars per hour to watch her children. The idea of paying six dollars so that she could just rest or go for a walk alone *never occurred to her*. In fact, she came to meetings only when she could drop her children off at her mother's house. If her mother wasn't able to look after the children for that hour, she missed the meeting.

"It may seem stupid to you Rosalie, but when I stopped myself before the binge and tried to figure out what was going on, all I could think of was that the baby was crying and that one of my twins needed changing. And then I realized that I needed a break! I just needed one. And then everything clicked. If I sat down and ate a cake or ordered in a pizza or Chinese food, it would come to the same six dollars it would cost me to have the girl down the block help me—so I asked myself, what am I doing standing here in front of the fridge? Getting ready to spoil all the work I've done for the last two weeks? Don't I deserve a break? And the minute I decided to call up the babysitter, I began to calm down."

"Great!" I said. "That's the way to go!" And her words gave me a lift that stayed with me through the day. Of course, if you had asked her before this: *Isn't your health and well-being worth six dollars?*, she would have said *Yes!* But she had to discover this on her own. It wasn't her natural way of thinking about things. People get caught up in life and lose perspective. They don't see what they're doing to themselves until it's too late—and then all they want is food because they've *let themselves* get to the point where that's the only answer; they've let themselves get so run-down and stressed out that they need the "instant solution" of a quick sugar fix, which only ends up adding to the problem because once they've started that binge, God only knows where it'll stop. The danger comes from the fact that bingeing is not about hunger and, after the first few bites, it's not even about taste. It's the mind that triggers the binge—and so only the mind can stop it. Once we've started, there's no end to what we can eat. That's why I say that the best way to stop a binge is not to begin it. It's so much harder to *regain* control once we've started eating—if only we could take this into account before that first cake or box of chocolates!

So I try to reason with myself when I feel a binge coming on. I take a step back no matter how I'm feeling and I ask myself: *Do you want to be happy tomorrow? To be happy! I forgot all about that!* I find myself thinking. *Am I hungry? Do I need it?* I argue with myself. *If you can get through the next hour without eating, you'll feel so good! What's a spoonful of ice cream going to do for you? Do you really think you're going to stop at a spoonful? Why should it be different this time—you'll eat a half gallon and you know how you'll end up feeling afterward*—and so the dialogue goes on.

I try to think of something to do that'll help me. And though I can't say I love exercise, sometimes I get on my bike and that reduces the stress. There are many ways you can make use of that moment when you haven't yet given in and binged. If you keep on practicing, you can isolate the overeating episodes to fewer and fewer occasions.

Three times in the last six months, I had a thought that shocked me: *Why don't you exercise now? You'll feel better.* And you have to understand that this thought—completely atypical of the old me—came to me in the middle of what would have been a three-cake crisis. Which goes to show you how, with time and patience, we can transform the most self-destructive aspects of our personality into a new way of life that sustains us.

"Sometimes I just need to eat," said a woman who'd been on maintenance a number of years. "So I make a huge pot of vegetable soup to keep myself from bingeing. The other night I was dying for a piece of cheesecake—so I had one bowl of soup after another and then I must have eaten about six or seven tangerines. I kept thinking of that cheesecake—but I wouldn't give in."

"Maybe you should have gone for the cake!" a young woman who'd lost about twenty pounds said to her. "I mean, that's what I've been doing. I sit down with a piece of cheesecake and a cup of coffee and I *stretch it out.* My husband said he's never seen anyone make a piece of cake last as long. I taste every mouthful— I eat it like a human being—and then I feel satisfied."

"The urge to eat is *Jaws,*" I said. "It's *anything!* The desire for a very special food is a different story—it can usually be satisfied with a portion of that food. And I recommend this as a solution because if not, many times we eat everything around that special food, and then at the end we eat what we wanted in the first place as well. A member told me that she wanted ice cream but she wouldn't let herself have it. She had a dietetic ice cream dessert, then sherbet and a low-calorie mousse pop, and then *finally* she had the ice cream. She could have just satisfied that craving—had it, gotten it over with, and then gone on from there."

A man who was almost at his goal weight added: "The same thing is true for me. I've learned that if I get really focused on something that I want, I'd better have it, no matter how high it is in calories. Otherwise I'm taking the chance that I'll go totally out of control—if not at that moment, then maybe a few days later."

"Sometimes you can do that," another woman said who'd just returned to Weight Watchers® after having been on a yearlong binge, "and sometimes you can't. It all depends on how much control you have at that particular time. There have been periods in my life when I can't even keep a box of graham crackers in the house—forget a cheesecake. It just sets me off."

Each of us must learn what works for us—there's no single right answer—and sometimes what works at one stage of the weight loss process is different from what works a year or two later. We're not the same people we were ten years ago, so there's no reason that our eating patterns should be the same.

"I broke down and binged on a box of chocolates this weekend," said a lovely young woman in one of my meetings, an accountant by profession. She was a lifetime member and had come back on a weekly basis because she regained five pounds and wanted to nip it in the bud. "I call chocolate my passion food—that's what made me start at Weight Watchers® to begin with. After a tough day at work last summer I found myself sitting on the couch surrounded by tinfoil wrappers from Kisses. They were everywhere. I must have gone through a few pounds of them, and when I saw all those wrappers I realized that I was totally out of control. Since I started coming here, I've learned to eat one chocolate brownie and call it quits. Or I can eat a small amount of chocolate pudding or have a slice of chocolate cake and stop. But when it comes to pure chocolate, I still go crazy and start bingeing. I thought I had more control than I did and that's what got me into trouble last weekend. So that's it—I'm keeping away from it because it's not worth it to me. I can't handle it."

"I would only add *for now*," I said. "Maybe you'll get more control as time goes on. You know, control is like a muscle—the more you exercise it, the stronger it becomes. In any case, you've tested your limits and have discovered what they are at this particular stage in the process. I've been at this for more years than I care to remember and I still keep tempting foods out of my house. That's one of *my* limits. It's a strength to know what you can and what you cannot do."

A New Idea: You Count!

A single woman in her thirties—I'll call her Just Two for reasons you'll see in a minute—had reached her goal weight and been on maintenance a long time when she fell into what I call a "bingette" instead of a binge, since the overeating was confined to one short session.

"What caused it?" I asked her when she brought it up at the meeting.

"Well, for one thing I'd had a hard day," she answered. "Our company has an exhibit at the gift show at the Coliseum and I was on my feet for hours, running around and trying to make sure that everything would go well. It wasn't only a question of making sure that everything was all right with our exhibits—we're an import-export company with displays of exotic gifts imported from the Far East. I also had to take notes on the displays arranged by our competitors and talk to various prospective customers. There was no time for my usual morning snack—I couldn't even find the apple and orange I always put into my handbag for an emergency. So I know my resistance was down by the end of the day.

"I knew that I didn't have much food in the apartment, so I dropped into a neighborhood restaurant for dinner on the way home and when I saw a woman at the next table eating French fries, I asked the waitress: 'Can I have two French fries? Just two?' I must have had such a pathetic look on my face that she brought me a whole plate—which was all I needed to start me off. I finished the fries and from that point on everything broke down. I went on to hamburgers, ice cream, the works."

"I understand how you felt," a woman in the group, a friend of hers, said in a kindly way. "But let's be honest—when you asked for just two French fries didn't you know she'd bring you the plate?"

"I really didn't," she said. "I told the waitress that she could charge me for a whole order but that she should just bring me two."

"So why didn't you say anything when she brought out the plate?"

"I didn't want to make a fuss—the fries were there already and I ate them."

Let's take this woman at her word. If only two fries had been brought out, *maybe* they would have been enough for her. Just a taste might have been what she craved—but her defenses were down. All day, she'd forgotten her own needs. Instead of preparing and bringing along snacks she could eat quickly during the day— no matter how hectic things get, everyone can grab five minutes here and there—she even forgot to bring along the fruit she always kept for emergencies.

Not only that, but she tells us that she ended up going to a restaurant because she didn't have much food in the house. All of which sounds to me like she didn't plan ahead or think about how exhausted she'd be at the end of the day. She knew what a strain the gift show would be and either she should have chosen a restaurant that had plenty of things on the menu she could eat or she should have come home to a fully prepared, low-calorie nourishing dinner ready to be heated.

But she'd been on maintenance a long time and one of the dangers of maintenance is that we sometimes get overconfident: she hadn't taken into consideration how the extra pressure would affect her eating—she'd taken her self-control for granted whereas in the beginning of her weight loss, she would have been more concerned. She wouldn't have been so casual about what was, after all, a challenge at work *that also meant a weight challenge.*

Okay, so even if the whole issue of the French fries hadn't come up, we can see that when she entered the restaurant she was in danger because she'd been driving on empty. And then she *compounded* the danger by letting the waitress decide the portion to be set in front of her—she'd asked for one thing but accepted another. Which, of course, is true for a lot of overweight people when they eat publicly.

Ah, you'll say, *why should this woman feel uncomfortable about eating in public? She was already on maintenance—she was already thin!* But the *reality* of the change, how a person looks after a major weight loss, takes a long time to sink in: the self-image of an overweight person, created over years, lingers on long after the weight is gone. We still move and act and think of ourselves as being the way we used to be. And overweight people do not want to make a fuss if they ask for a salad without dressing and then get one dripping with oil. They don't want to call attention to themselves. They're often shy about sending the food back if they've ordered a dry English muffin and they get one heavily buttered. *People are going to look at me,* they think, *and wonder why is* she *making a commotion about butter?* They haven't yet got to the stage where they can say: *We* do *count and what we want* is *important. We* are *entitled* to ask for what we want.

In this case, insisting on getting what she wanted might have

helped Just Two through a difficult meal. Or it might be that she
was just ready to binge and looking for an excuse. Either way,
she'd learned useful habits during the time she'd been on maintenance. One of them was going right back on program after a
binge—and that saved her.

"The binge cost me three pounds," Just Two said—but over
the years she'd developed the right attitude toward those pounds.
She didn't ignore them, because she knew how easily the pounds
can creep up. "The question you asked at one of the meetings kept
running through my mind, Rosalie: *Are we talking about three
pounds or are we talking about* THE FIRST *three pounds?*" But
she didn't let herself become desperate over them, either. She knew
desperation just leads to more eating.

Just Two had had a hard day and she'd learned to put yesterday
behind her. But there are times when the problem is long-term and
then the solution has to be long-term.

Take the very impressive case of someone I really admire. I'll
call her my Painted Lady because she's the Virginia Kelly type—
she's heavily made up and always wears lots and lots of jewelry.
She's the salt of the earth and a very religious Catholic to boot.
With a great deal of willpower and a lot of hard work she lost
forty pounds—and you have to remember that for a woman in
her sixties this is more difficult since the metabolism slows down.
In this woman's case especially, the medication she was on (an
essential one) slowed down her weight loss even more. So those
forty pounds represented a long, hard battle—that she won.

Stage one. She'd learned how to cope with food and how to
integrate her new eating patterns into her life and then her life
changed, or I should say that problems already there heated up.
Everything escalated. Her husband had severe diabetes and his
sugar had to be continually monitored. Finally, things got so bad
that he had to have his leg amputated. The new level of care he
needed, the medical bills, the added concern all began to push her
back toward food.

"My husband is a smoker—I guess I should say a compulsive
smoker. His smoking makes me crazy because I know what it does
to his health. But I feel terrible when I fight with him about it
because he's been through hell and the cigarettes relax him," she

said at one meeting. "But if I bottle it up inside, it also makes me feel crazy and I eat like there's no tomorrow."

"So why don't you try reasoning with him instead of fighting?" an "idealist" in the group asked.

"Ha! Go reason with a block of wood," The Painted Lady answered. "Yesterday, I had to open all the windows in the house just to get some air to breathe. But there's no talking to him. With diabetes, if he gets excited his sugar goes up. It's not good for him—but it's hard to remember that when he's smoking like a chimney or when I catch him eating something that's not good for him. He always says he's sorry, but then he goes back and does the same thing all over again when he gets a chance. He drives me crazy!"

"You remember that old line: *A husband is a man who'll stand by you through all the troubles you would not have had if you hadn't married him?*" a woman put in.

"I heard it about a wife!" a man in the group said.

"Same difference," I said. "The bottom line is that it's very hard when you're dealing with someone you love who's sick." I thought of all the husbands and wives who come to the meetings grieving over the illness of their spouses. "That's the problem here: we're dealing with an ongoing situation. You're always going to be worried about his health and his smoking—you just have to make your mind up to that. So you have to figure out a strategy."

"What kind of a strategy?" she asked.

"Well, first of all, when you're faced with a problem like this one, a life situation that's very difficult, you have to ask yourself: *When you get up every morning, are you at your best or are you tired, stressed out, worn out already?* Any strategy you use, first of all, has to be directed toward *you* taking care of *you*." I paused for a minute to let this sink in. "You don't have to tell me this now—but I would just like you to see if you can think of three things you've done for yourself in the last week."

"I can tell you since you know I've been bingeing anyway," The Painted Lady answered. "I bought myself my favorite Godiva chocolates and—do you want to hear what else?"

"Besides food, I mean. What did you *do* for yourself?"

She thought about it but she didn't say a word.

"You see what I mean? It's enough that your husband is in trouble—why do you have to join him? If you keep taking care of yourself with food—which in my book is the same as not taking care of yourself at all—you'll end up joining your husband at the doctor's office. And even if you're lucky and keep your health, do you really want to become obese?"

I paused again because I wanted my question to make an impression on her. I'd mentioned obesity because that's where she was heading and it was important for her to realize it. "Besides, if you don't stay healthy, how are you going to take care of him?" I asked. "If you can't think of *yourself*, maybe thinking of *him* will make you take care of yourself!"

I reminded her of our rule, *A BANKRUPT PERSON CAN'T GIVE ANYTHING TO ANYONE*—it's a rule I never tire of repeating because so many times, overweight people give and give and give until there's nothing left and so they turn to food. I've seen this in so many different situations—the players and settings may be different but the script is the same. It's such a major problem that I wish I could be there, whispering over their shoulder like the Devil they need: Just Say No! *Turn down that good cause, or that neighbor who needs a ride, or that friend who just wants your help for five minutes—those five minutes will turn into an afternoon you need for yourself—mark my words! Take a nap or go for a walk instead. You need it!*

The Painted Lady had to learn to be a good wife without destroying herself.

"You don't understand," she said. "Forget about *three* things I've done—I almost didn't get to the meeting today. I don't have any time between my kids—they come over with their kids to cheer my husband up. It's a lot of work to—"

"Just wait a minute," I interrupted her. "Someone *has to give way*. Dr. Joyce Brothers once said, *There is a rule in sailing that the more maneuverable ship should give way to the less maneuverable craft. And this is a good rule to follow in human relationships as well.* When it comes to these meetings, you have to be like a battleship. The time you put aside for them should be sacred. It should be a "given"—no questions asked. We're talking about one hour now. If I told you it would take one hour of your week to help keep you thin all the other hours of your week, wouldn't that seem like a great trade-off, a super deal? And when you consider all the problems, physical as well as emotional, that being overweight entails, the deal gets better and better."

Taking care of yourself is nothing more or less than loving yourself—and this is the number one way to prevent a binge. As Lucille Ball often said when asked about the secret of her success: *Love yourself first and everything else falls into line. You have to really love yourself to get anything done in this world.*

Some Practical Ways to Nourish Yourself— Without Food!

There are many different ways that this new attitude toward ourselves can become a practical reality. Sometimes it's giving ourselves the time we need to regroup, relax, recover from a stressful day; sometimes it's spending the money on healthy but expensive food we normally would think twice about buying. Sometimes it's just standing up for ourselves, putting our own needs before others.

A working mother who was slowly getting control over her eating said, "My kids tried to talk me into a dog—but I know who'd end up taking care of it once the novelty wears off. So I said to them, 'You can choose between me and the dog!' And you know what? The only one who voted for me was my husband!"

"You must be doing something for him that you don't do for them!" a woman joked and everyone laughed.

"So what happened?" I asked.

"I guess my house is not a democracy because we didn't get the dog. The old me would have given in and been out there walking the dog before work or running to the vet with it when it got sick. But now I'm into taking care of myself and I told them I didn't want to even think about one more obligation. And I know the kids sense a change."

"Actually, you're giving them a valuable lesson," said an older woman who'd been on maintenance a long time. "When I first started working, I took a night job because I didn't want to leave my kids during the day. I served dinner, I cleaned up, and then I left for work. I did it willingly and loved taking care of my family. But within six months, I noticed I was getting worn out. I used to come home and find dishes, pots, and pans waiting for me in the sink. At first I never bothered asking them to clean up because I thought they would see what they should do themselves, but nobody does anything unless they're asked!"

"Nobody is clairvoyant," I put in. "When they see dishes are in the sink, they think that's just the way it is."

"What I learned," the older woman went on, "is that instead of yelling, 'You never help me and you're such a slob!', it's easy to ask directly for help. And to ask again—and again, until your family understands that every time they leave a plate in the sink, they're leaving it for someone else. Why sit around feeling sorry for yourself when you can change things if you just open your mouth?"

"I think women especially have been taught not to express their anger directly so they eat to swallow their feelings," a young woman added.

But there are also plenty of men who have trouble saying NO— and we're not only talking about setting limits for other people, but sometimes, when we're driven and workaholic, we have to learn to say NO to ourselves. For many disciplined people, food is the only area where they loosen up—and before they can change that, they have to find other ways they can "give in" to themselves.

One man in my group, a stockbroker, joined only because they had to scoop him up off the office floor after he'd had a heart attack. His doctor terrified him—either he started losing weight or else. His wife, also very overweight, had joined him to give him moral support. "I'd come back to the office to work after a long day and the only thing that kept me at my desk was food. I'd order in pizza or Chinese food and milkshakes—and that was *after* a dinner with a client at a vegetarian health food restaurant."

"Sometimes money costs too much!" I said.

"It's not just the money. It's the challenge. The sense of satisfaction I get from doing well," he answered.

"Then maybe you need to find other ways of getting satisfaction. Things less stressful," I added.

"For example?" he asked.

"That's something you'll have to discover for yourself. It's different for everyone, but what I've learned is that what I do to nourish myself in non-food ways is the most valuable use I could possibly make of my time. But most of us are too pressured, too harried—so we turn to food. It's easy. It takes about one minute— you can start eating as quickly as it takes you to open the fridge or go from your office to a local coffee shop. And it means you don't have to deal with your feelings. You're blissed out with all that food."

One woman told the group that when her sister called, she could tell just by the sound of her voice if she'd been bingeing— there was a faraway, everything-is-right-with-the-world sound to it that gave her away.

"I'll bet that was me!" said a young woman who ran a busy household and at the same time held down a stressful job working for the Emergency Medical Services as a paramedic. "I see what being overweight does to people every day and you'd think that would keep me from bingeing! We have an article pasted up on our bulletin board at the hospital that says three hundred thousand Americans die every year of weight-related diseases—three hundred thousand! That alone should keep me thin."

"Well, fear only goes so far," I said. "It's a good motivator but you need a carrot to go along with the stick."

"Please! If I hear the word *carrot* I'll get sick!" she laughed. "This was an ice cream week—ice cream is my thing. I put on two point four pounds. I tried your advice of asking myself *What do I really want now?*—only I waited until after the Ben and Jerry's to ask myself the question."

Everyone laughed.

"Better late than never," I said.

"No, I really did," she said. "First I sat down and forced myself to write everything I'd eaten—and the list was scary. I figured it out and then added up the calories just to make myself realize what I was doing. That put an end to this lingering thought, *Maybe I'll just wait one more day to end this binge.*"

"That's a great technique," I added. "In general I like writing things down because something takes over when you start to write.

If you really try to be honest with yourself, sometimes you can surprise yourself with what comes out on the page. Your unconscious takes over and you learn things about yourself that you didn't know before."

"One thing that came up was that I felt guilty because I'm away from the kids so much. So when I'm home, they get away with murder because I have a hard time saying NO! to them. Instead, I just eat."

"Well, you're not out dancing or shopping all day—you're working for their sake as well as yours!" an older woman in the group pointed out in a sympathetic voice. "And it's very stressful work, too. Not everybody could stand the pressure of all those medical emergencies."

"Still, that's how I feel. I guess I wish I could raise them the way I was raised."

"It's better to write out those feelings than to eat them in the form of chocolate and cake," I said. "At least you know what you're feeling—*plus* you've figured out a great way to help put the brakes on. You should keep that list of everything you've eaten and write on the bottom of it how you felt afterwards. And the next time you want to binge, maybe reading it through first will help."

In the Middle of a Binge? These Tips Will Save You

Let me sum up with a few helpful steps to take once the binge has begun—because there's no reason that you have to eat yourself to the bitter end of every binge. As I see it, it's like fighting with someone you love. One word leads to another and before you know it you're in the midst of a battle without wanting to be there! But just as there are many chances to stop the escalation of the fight between that first angry word and the final *I'll never talk to you again!*—the same is true of a binge. We don't want it to start. But once it's started, we can try to put an end to it before it's done too much damage. The longer it goes on, the harder it is to stop.

If, as you're devouring the chocolate cake (and before you ask yourself *What's next?*), just one of these techniques puts a stop to the eating, then you're way ahead of the game.

The first step is very important: CALM DOWN! The worse you make yourself feel, the longer the binge will go on.

- Listen to the thoughts running through your mind and put an immediate stop to all criticism and harsh self-rebuke. Have some kindness for yourself.
- Make the best of it.
- Change the location. There's a saying in real estate: *the three most important factors are* location, location, and location. The same thing is often true of bingeing; the place you're in can affect you. When you're sitting in the kitchen or near the TV or in any place where you normally eat and notice that you've begun to nibble—a bite of this, a taste of that—get up and go somewhere else before a binge develops. This is even more important once the binge has begun.
- Change what you're doing—that can also help to break a pattern. We're such creatures of habit that certain places and activities almost automatically send us to food, since that's our association.
- Delay. When you eat, it takes about twenty minutes for the stomach to signal the brain that all is well, twenty minutes for the effects of the food to be fully felt. Try to remember that fact and see if you can wait out the desire to binge.
- Distract yourself. Even in the middle of a binge, if you distract yourself with another activity it allows you to think and see the big picture. When I want to binge all I see is the great food. How much I want it. What it's going to taste like. How much I have to have it—that's the little picture. But the big picture is the bloated stomach. The empty boxes and wrappers. The extra weight. The clothes that don't fit. The worry about what to wear to work the next day. The feelings of guilt and hopelessness. If you're eating because of happiness—CELEBRATE! Buy yourself something nice. Go to the theater. Spread the happiness. Call somebody. Go roller skating. Be active.

And if you're miserable, you can try helping someone, too.

You can watch a movie. And if you're going to eat anyway, despite all of this, try to start with appropriate foods. It depends on your mood and the taste and the texture of the food that satisfies you. For anger you might want something bulky, crunchy, chewy—popcorn, carrots. For comfort, it might be that you're looking for a food that slides down. Hot or cold vegetable soup, Jell-O, sugar-free chocolate pudding, a fruit milkshake.

- If you have a specific food in mind, go for it. Don't eat *around* what you really want: *start*, don't finish with it—but make it hard to overeat. Buy only one portion of the food. Or eat it in a public place. A small portion of ice cream eaten in an ice cream shop is a treat. A half gallon straight out of the carton, eaten quickly, is a binge.

- If you've started eating a food that you normally have in the house, like cereal or graham crackers, you can also make the overeating harder. If you are holding a box of cereal in your hand, you will consume the entire box—trust me. Instead put a small amount of cereal in a bowl and put the box away before you start eating. If you want more, get the box out, and pour some more into the bowl. Force yourself to go back each time. You are buying time to think and to impose a level of control.

- No self-punishment. If you were planning to have bread and a hamburger for dinner, have the bread, have the hamburger. Trying to "make up" for the binge by skipping a planned meal will only lead you back to bingeing again.

- Don't cut back the next day. You need to treat yourself better than ever after a binge.

- Remind yourself of your success. Don't let a single binge make you forget all the hard-won victories you've had during your time on program. It takes strength and courage to fight the need to eat on a daily basis—appreciate your progress. Be proud of your effort.

- And finally, GET RIGHT BACK ON THE PROGRAM. The successful people are the ones who can pick themselves up after a binge and continue as if nothing happened. What's the use of harping on mistakes? There's an old Chinese saying: *The best time to plant a tree was twenty years ago. The second-best time is now.*

- Let me conclude with some words from Julia Child, of all people—someone who knows all about the pleasures of food. *Life,* she said, *is the best binge.* The next time we want to binge, instead of turning to food, why not give life a chance?

CHAPTER SEVEN

The Scale—Facing the Music

If you keep one eye on the goal, that only leaves you one
eye to look at the road.

—Old Saying

Discovery consists of looking at the same thing as everyone
else and thinking something different.

—Albert Szent-Gyorgyi, American biochemist

The scale is only a piece of machinery, right? (Wrong!) What is
it? Some springs and metal with numbers under a glass and an
arrow pointing to them—true or false? (False!)

Let me begin by stating a surprising fact. THE SCALE CAN
LIE—on a day-to-day basis, and sometimes from week to week.

Yes, though most of us think of the scale as a completely objective tool, the numbers can be your worst enemy when taken out
of context. You can't argue with the numbers, you say. It's the
last court of appeal. It's the be-all and end-all, the bottom line—
but we've all had times when this hasn't been true.

Sometimes you can cheat the scale (*Ah, you think, I've gotten
away with that box of doughnuts! Thank God!*) and sometimes
the scale can cheat you (*What? A whole week of walking and
staying on the program and I've gained a pound! I didn't deserve
that!*). In the short term, this isn't the way to measure your success.
Why is that?

Hold that question! as I say at the meetings. *We're coming to
that!* First, let me pose the riddle raised by a woman who attended

meetings on and off for the last year, a celebrity whose name I won't mention (suffice it to say that she's a household name). "I was so nervous before I weighed in this morning that I almost left my pocketbook in the ladies' room—" (and this from a lady who was cool, calm, and collected before cameras on national TV). "I had no idea this week which way it was going to go and until the last minute I kept praying, *Please God! Just don't let me gain!*"

"So, how did you do?" I asked.

"I lost two pounds and I feel really happy, really vindicated!" She smiled—and let me say that it was the first time I'd seen her smile since she started coming. "That brings the grand total up to twenty pounds. I'm not ashamed to tell the group that I'm now one hundred and sixty-two gorgeous pounds."

Everybody applauded and the truth is, she needed to lose those twenty pounds at this point in her career—she's gone the book and lecture route. Professionally, it was a do-or-die step for her. She went on, though, to make an interesting observation which I've heard in one form or another from many people:

"But as I sit here now I can't help thinking that the same number I saw today and that made me so happy—one hundred and sixty-two pounds—would have made me miserable just five years ago. I would have been horrified. The difference is that now I'm seeing it on my way down whereas before I was seeing it on my way up."

"The difference is you're in *control* now," I emphasized. "So I guess it's not really about the numbers after all, or maybe not *just* about the numbers." I wanted everyone in the room to think beyond the moment of weighing-in, hoping that sooner or later they would be free from the tyranny of the scale. "162 lbs. on the way up was a *symbol* of out-of-control eating. Now 162 lbs. on the way down is a *symbol* of hard work and success. The number is a symbol and *only* a symbol. If you forget that, you're in its power."

If this is true, why was our celebrity so nervous before she got on the scale? She must have known she was in control. She must have been doing something right all week to have lost two pounds; why did she need the scale to tell her that? And let me add another twist to the plot: let's say she hadn't lost any weight that week, what then? What would that have meant? Worse: what if she'd gained a pound, a pound and a half? Would that have invalidated all her hard work? How many times does it happen that you know you've been in control and the scale goes up? It's easy to say, *Are you going to let a machine control your entire perception of yourself?* But the truth is you're only human! You were looking forward to seeing the *results* of all your hard work. After a week filled with temptations that you've resisted, you want that reflected in a lower number on the scale.

But there are any number of reasons it doesn't always work that way. It could be that you wear heavier clothes one week. It could be that your body is retaining more roughage. It could be something as simple as having eaten a very salty meal the night before and you're retaining water (you'll lose this kind of weight right away). Medication you are on sometimes plays a part—there are many medications that affect the metabolism such as strong antibiotics or steroids, while antidepressants increase appetite. The time of the month is often a very important factor. Extra jewelry. You weigh in at a different hour. Sometimes the body resists letting go of those extra pounds and it just takes an extra push, another week or two, to tip the scale in your favor. The list could go on forever—it's like the old saying: *There are lies, there are damned lies, and there are statistics.*

I'm not saying that you should immediately attribute a weight gain to one or more of these reasons. If you've gained weight, you should first of all go over the foods you've eaten during the week and *double check on their values.* It could be that you discover a particular food has a higher calorie count than you knew. I've had a member who was shocked to discover that pasta is equivalent to bread! This is an intelligent, hardworking, honest lady who loves pasta—I call her my Pasta Queen. But she had no idea of how to work it into her meals. She'd never thought of measuring it before she came to Weight Watchers®: "It seemed like such a healthy food to me!" *Oh come on,* you might think, *who doesn't know that?* But the truth is that there are surprises in store for almost everyone who decides to eat more *consciously,* to know the effect of everything they put into their mouths.

Then there are the little tastes—a bite of this, a spoonful of that, a handful, a nibble, a lick, a swig, a sliver, a mouthful, a sip. It's not just in the world of money that little sums add up into big ones.

If you've been keeping a record of everything you've eaten, you should review the record carefully and see if you've gone over your limits. If you haven't been tracking your food, you should make sure to track it the following week. But once you've come to the conclusion that you're doing everything correctly and still you've gained a small amount of weight or haven't lost weight for one week you should FORGET IT! I have seen those disappointments ruin morale, lead to out-of-control eating, and cause people who were doing so well to give up! One of the reasons we focus on the numbers so intently is that we don't realize that in weight loss, the means are more important than the end. Once we master the process, the numbers take care of themselves.

In the long run, we get what we deserve. If you overeat, it will catch up to you. And a week on program is like money in the bank—sooner or later it will pay interest. One week we gain a pound for no reason. Another week, we lose a pound—again seemingly for no reason. We think in terms of the last few days, the last week, and forget about the big picture. It reminds me of something Jack Benny once said when accepting an award: "I don't deserve this. But then, I don't deserve my arthritis, either!" Sooner or later, it all evens out, it all balances.

But the bottom line is, long run or short, we don't *need* the scale to tell us how we've done. We know if we've overeaten; we know if we've been exercising. The fear, the anxiety about stepping onto that machine comes from not trusting ourselves. We want a reality check outside ourselves, which is not a bad thing, either. It's like what the former Mayor of New York, Ed Koch, always used to ask: *How am I doing?* We need a voice that says: You're doing a great job! But the scale can not always be that voice.

A woman I'll call Nothing Throws Me, a former airline stewardess, refused to play the numbers game. "I just want my health back," she confided to me privately, because her extra pounds were making it hard for her to walk. One day before the meeting started, she came up to show me photos of her new great-grandchild, a beautiful little girl of four months. "I'm a mother all over again, Rosalie."

"You get the best of both worlds," I said, thinking of my own grandchildren.

"Well," she remarked, "in this case the child will be living with me from now on. That's where I was last week—I flew to Minnesota to bring her home."

"Sounds like a big job," I told her, concerned about her overtaxing herself. I know the kind of person she is: she's always there for other people; she's active in charity work; an elderly neighbor depends on her. She's even worried about me—last year she discovered some new, low calorie, Kosher-for-Passover food and gave it to me as a gift. I know the tendency many overweight people have to take on more than they can handle, and I was hoping that Nothing Throws Me knew what she was doing. It turned out that she did.

"My granddaughter got mixed up with someone who, when he found out he was going to be a father, wanted her to have an abortion. I'm proud of her because when the time came, she couldn't bring herself to do it. And she's only sixteen. Rosalie, what makes things harder is that the father is black and my daughter married into a family that—well, don't get me started about them. To make a long story short, that's why I missed the meeting last week. My granddaughter had no one to turn to but me so I got on the next plane to Minnesota."

A few weeks later an interesting fact about her trip emerged. Despite everything she had to do, Nothing Throws Me made the time to attend a Weight Watchers® meeting in Minnesota. When she weighed in, though, she was horrified to discover that she'd gained five pounds. "You know, hearing that news from strangers made it even worse. I've been coming here so long that I think of this as my Weight Watchers™ family. What made it doubly hard to take was that I was expecting good news. Even though it was impossible to stick to my usual routines, I thought I'd managed well. I had no desire to eat BEFORE I went on that scale. But the moment I got off it, this crazy voice in my head kept saying, *You've gained all that weight and you haven't even gotten to eat what you wanted. If you're going to gain weight already, at least have some ice cream, for God's sake. How many years has it been since you've had a banana split?* It went on and on that way. The people in Minnesota told me I could allow a one- to two-pound variation from the scale I regularly used, but that still left me with a three-pound weight gain. I was so demoralized! But I didn't give in. I had a little extra fruit, but nothing else."

"You had the banana without the split?" There was laughter. "What stopped you?" I asked.

"I just kept remembering a saying you'd quoted once, Rosalie: *Don't quit ten minutes before the miracle!* I *knew* I'd been good: why should I allow that one weigh-in to ruin all my hard work?"

"Great!" I said.

"And the payoff was that when I got home, not only hadn't I gained a pound, but I actually had lost two and a half."

"It was probably just a lot of what I call water weight," Rosalie said. "Maybe the new foods you were eating affected you."

"You deserve a banana split!" someone joked, to which I replied, "Please! She's got much more than that. She's got her self-respect!"

In the face of her weight disaster—not to mention her family problems—Nothing Throws Me persisted. She felt discouraged, but she simply refused to give in. I read a quotation from Calvin Coolidge which exactly describes the kind of mental attitude necessary for this kind of success: *Nothing in the world can take the place of persistence. Talent will not. Nothing is more common that unsuccessful men with talent. Genius will not. Unrewarded genius is almost a proverb. Education will not. The world is full of educated derelicts. Persistence and determination alone are omnipotent.*

Dealing with Discouragement

Nothing-Throws-Me was dealing with an unusual situation, but the principle that kept her from getting discouraged is one that applies across the board. If you have faith in yourself and in what you're doing, the truth is that nothing can shake you. And if you're a pessimist, even if everything is going your way, you can turn your triumph into a defeat. How many times, for example, have

I heard people moan *I only lost one pound this week*. They came to the meeting thinking that they'd lost at least three pounds, maybe five, so naturally when the arrow just moved one pound down it felt like a disaster. Another person, seeing that one-pound loss, will be thrilled and say: *Thank God! Another pound off*. And we're talking about the same pound here.

Of course I understand why people become discouraged: they're working hard, they have fifty or more pounds to lose, and it seems like it's taking forever. The old saying, *If you lose a pound a week, that's fifty-two pounds in a year* doesn't do it for them because they are concentrating on what's wrong, not on what's right. It comes back to faith. You know how the joke goes—*The trouble with pessimism is that it doesn't work!*

Sometimes the weight loss seems unbearably slow because the *last time* around, the person lost weight more quickly. It's important to remember that most successful, long-term members have gone through the process of losing the weight and gaining it all back at least once or twice before they finally learn how to keep it off forever. They were what I call my "successful failures" before they became successes: they learned how to turn failure into feedback, how to learn from their mistakes. They have the advantage of being stronger people as a result. When they finally reach their goal weight with all that experience, they remain at it. The *disadvantage* is that the third or fourth time around, the weight loss slows down. Over the years, I've see this happen again and again and we have to be ready for it. It's something we can't change, so we just have to take it into account and change our expectations. It's healthier to have lower expectations than to be disappointed week after week.

Okay, so we've lost a pound this time around whereas last time, given the same amount of food and effort, we would have lost three. So we've lost a pound while the man or woman sitting next to us has lost five. It's human nature to make these kinds of comparisons. The trick is not to let this get us down, to defeat us. Instead of pressuring ourselves, instead of hurrying up the weight loss by being "better"—too much pressure is unhealthy—we must learn to rejoice in other successes. Opening your closet and having clothes to wear, not having eaten your way up a size, are successes.

That feeling you have when you go to sleep at the end of a good day on the program—that's success.

The struggle along the way, the effort you put into that struggle, is a kind of success which we must also learn to appreciate. It reminds me of something Norman Lear said during an interview for *Parade* magazine. "Throughout the American scene—television, sports, government—the message seems to be that life is made up of winners and losers. If you are not number one or in the top five, you have failed. *There doesn't seem to be any reward for simply succeeding at the level of doing one's best.* Success is how you collect your minutes. You spend millions of minutes to reach one triumph, one moment, then you spend maybe a thousand minutes enjoying it. If you are unhappy through those millions of minutes, what good are the thousand minutes of triumph? It doesn't equate. Life is made of small pleasures. Good eye contact over the breakfast table with your wife. A moment of touching with a friend. Happiness is made of those tiny successes. The big ones come too infrequently. If you don't have all of those zillions of tiny successes, the big ones don't mean anything. If there is one thing I want my children to learn from me, it is to take pleasure in life's daily small successes. It is the most important thing I've learned."

I asked my group members this question: "Imagine that there is no such thing in the world as a scale. Let's pretend it hadn't been invented. How would you know that you are losing weight, that your body is changing, that your attitudes and habits are changing?"

"A thinner face!" one woman called out immediately. "I wouldn't give a damn what the scale said if I had a thinner face."

"Loose clothes," someone sighed. "And I don't mean muumuus. I mean jeans or a dress that just hung on you."

"Yes, just being able to wear a belt!" I added. "In my fat life, I never tucked in my blouse. I always had to wear a pullover or an overblouse or something to hide my waist. Now I have a whole collection of belts. I love them! Whenever I find a belt that matches my outfit, I buy it."

"I know I'm doing well when I have more energy," a woman

holding a sleeping child said. "When I had fifty extra pounds on, I never wanted to leave the house."

"Loose jewelry," another woman said, holding up hands covered with rings.

"Eating one slice of pizza instead of four!" a man I'll call The Pizza Lover said. "After the first slice it's not about hunger anyway!"

"Learning to eat in a restaurant and leave food on my plate. It's better to pay for it with money than with extra pounds!"

"I watch the video from my son's wedding," another woman said. "I could look at myself again and again in the dress I wore. If I hadn't really changed, I never could have worn a dress like that one."

"For me, just being able to cross my legs for the first time in five years is a sign that I'm on the way," a woman who had lost fifty pounds said with pride. Can any fluctuation of a pound or two on the scale take away that pride?

That's why it's so important, so vital for people to develop their own criteria for success! It will keep them from out-of-control eating when the scale disappoints them, as sooner or later it disappoints everyone at one time or another.

Sometimes, the "sign" of change has nothing to do with the body directly. An example of this is a woman I'll call Don't-Step-On-My-Toes. She'd led a very active life during the years she was an assistant for an important elected official, but after her retirement she put on a great deal of weight. It was hard for her to rechannel her energies and skills. She had more time to brood over problems which she used to forget about in the course of a busy, challenging day.

She'd always been "on the borderline," but now her steady weight gain put her into a whole new weight range. Finally, very high blood pressure scared her into taking notice of what was happening to her body and during the next year and a half, she lost more than thirty pounds. For the last two months, though, she'd been on what's called a "plateau"—that is, she'd remained at the same weight although she was sticking to the program and had continued to exercise. What was unusual about her, though, was that she truly wasn't discouraged—just the opposite. The fact that her weight loss had helped bring down her blood pressure put her in a very positive frame of mind. "I feel grateful that the dizzy spells have let up. I thank God every morning that I was spared a stroke," she said with so much feeling in her voice that you could see she meant every word. Her positive attitude also enabled her to appreciate other changes taking place as a result of her weight loss, changes that she wouldn't have seen if she'd been blinded by those numbers on the scale.

"I'll give you an example from something that happened last week," she said in response to my question about life in a scale-less world. "I became *furious* with my son-in-law—we'd helped him out all through his years in law school and now, when we need his help buying a summer house, he lets two or three days go by before he returns our calls. The old me would have just sat down with cake and candy to calm down. This time, Rosalie, instead of eating, I left a message on his voice mail that must have made his ears burn—believe me, he called back and apologized the same day. I'd shocked everyone by behaving in a way that just wasn't *me*. And I think that the person who was most shocked of all was me.

"You know, before this I knew that when I ate, I used to let everything slide—the house, my appearance, everything from thank-you notes to answering calls was put *on hold*. But I never realized before that my eating also affected the way I dealt with people. I guess it was easier to eat than to tell them how I felt and I've felt proud of myself all week."

The way she controlled her food in response to a highly charged emotional situation was an important indicator of change for this woman. She gave herself credit for new behavior and she deserved that credit every bit as much as if the number on the scale had gone down ten pounds! *New behavior* is the name of the weight-loss game, because—*RULE! IF YOU KEEP DOING WHAT YOU'VE DONE, YOU'LL KEEP GETTING WHAT YOU'VE GOT.*

Alternatives to the Numbers Game

Behavior change can take many different forms and it's important to remember that it doesn't have to be earth-shattering to be meaningful. Take the example of a woman in her late forties who worked in a private high school in Brooklyn—I'll call her The School Secretary. Part of what's often called the "sandwich generation", caught between demanding parents and demanding children, she held down two jobs in order to put her daughters through college and at the same time help out her elderly parents, who were having financial problems. She'd been having her ups and downs at weight loss, but the overall picture was good: she'd managed to take off twenty pounds and keep them off during a nine-month period. Slow but steady, which is always a good sign in terms of future maintenance.

Her constant complaint was that it was taking so long. "If I lose a pound one week, a single pound, I never manage to lose anything the next week. That's the way it's been going since I started," she said at one meeting. "And the minute I eat a little bit more—I'm not talking about cake now, but if I just have an extra piece of chicken or too much fruit, I can forget losing anything for the week. It's just not fair—it's not fair!"

I suggested that she try *graphing* her weight loss, a technique that's helped many others (including myself) at low points in the struggle. A graph can be a useful tool because once you actually *see* your pattern of weight loss in front of you, it's easier to understand it and to get a sense of what's coming up in the future. The pound or two you lost or didn't lose on the scale is immediately put into visual perspective on a sheet of graph paper. It gives you a better sense of where you're coming from by *visually* reminding you of all the pounds you've taken off: those twenty pounds look like a mountain on the graph—maybe (in School Secretary's case) a gently sloping mountain with no steep valleys or plunging ravines, but a mountain all the same, and an impressive achievement.

She tried it and it helped for a while, but possibly because every other area of her life was so pressured, she just couldn't relax her frustrations and fears when it came to her weight. Her slow rate of loss still remained a sore spot, and on the day I took up the subject of the scale, she was in a particularly bad mood. She'd come to the meeting looking grim, with a very unhappy and nervous expression. And when another member, The Beauty Parlor Owner, objected to my questioning the scale, she nodded her head in strong agreement.

"All that doesn't work for me," The Beauty Parlor Owner said. "The only way I *know* I've lost weight is when the numbers go down. Otherwise it's too easy to lie to myself—I see a lot of that. I know a woman who goes to a gym a few times a week and does a full workout—the weights, the machines, the whole bit. She buys only health foods and hasn't touched sugar in a very long time. What does she think, health food doesn't have any calories? There are fat rabbits, too, you know!"

Everyone laughed and The School Secretary asked, "How does she look?"

"She looks *terrible*. She has three chins and she's carrying at least forty extra pounds. Whenever she comes in, she asks the girl who does her hair: 'What do you think?,' pointing at herself with pride. 'How do you like the figure?' And what's the girl supposed to say?"

"Well, what's wrong with that if she's happy?" someone asked.

"She's a young woman and she's putting on more and more weight all the time—where do you think she's heading? And how happy could she be if she's always talking about how well she's doing? She wouldn't have to make such a big deal about it if she didn't know the truth deep down. That's why she never steps on a scale. We all play along, but she's kidding herself."

"That's the other side of the coin," I remarked. "If that young woman got on the scale and it told her she was gaining weight week after week, believe me, she could be sure it was no accident. It would force her to see that she was doing something wrong. It's just as big a mistake to discard the scale entirely as it is to get obsessed by it. What I'm talking about here is understanding its limitations. I used to get on the scale every single morning and whatever the number was would set my mood for the whole day. If I'd gained, no matter what good things happened to me that day, I'd feel depressed; and if I'd lost, I had this sense of elation all day. No matter what. Now I weigh in once a week and I've come to the point where if I know I've been trying honestly and haven't overeaten, I won't be upset if the scale doesn't show this."

"Maybe that's because you've already lost all your weight," The School Secretary said. "For me, it's much harder."

"No, that's *how* I lost the weight," I answered honestly. "When I still had a long way to go, I decided in my gut: I don't care how long it takes—that's it. If I'm in this for the rest of my life, what's the difference if I reach my goal in May or April or June—or even *next* May, April, or June? As long as I do what I have to do, sooner or later I *know* it will work. So, I just told myself—*I'll be there when I get there,* and that was the end of a lifetime of torturing myself on the scale. I finally realized that I was setting myself up for disaster the other way. They say you either learn or you don't. I learned—it took me forever, but I finally, finally, finally got it into my head that, during the whole weight loss process, there had to be satisfactions besides a lower number. And I'm sure if you think about it carefully," I turned to The School Secretary, "you can come up with at least one success apart from the scale, some new habit, some victory you've had this week that shows you you're on the right path."

"This hasn't been such a great week for me," The School Secretary said.

"All right," I said, "during the last month then. I'm not asking you to share it with us—I really don't mean to put you on the spot. I'm only asking you to think about it when you go home, because I know it will help you."

"Yes, it's true there are some things I'm happy about in terms of my weight," she answered. "My clothes are fitting better, I notice that, and I haven't binged for a long time."

"You see what I mean?" I said.

"Why don't you tell her about the fire drill?" a friend of hers called out.

"Oh, that," The School Secretary said. "I forgot all about it."

"Come on, let's hear!" I urged her, wanting her to break out of a prison of pessimism and defeatism that she'd built for herself.

"Well, usually my workplace is safe for me since I don't like to eat at my desk. But when there are fire drills—and they never give any warning for them—there are always two hours I have to be out of the building. Somehow I'd gotten into the habit of dropping by a local pizzeria for diet soda. That's what I always told myself—these were never planned eating sessions. I never told myself that I was about to let myself go. It was just that I like the people at the pizzeria—they've known me for years—so it was easy to kid myself into believing that I was just going there to kill time. Plus, I'd always *start out* with just diet soda—but after a while I'd relax and have a slice of pizza to go with the soda—after all, there's nothing wrong with pizza. You can have a slice and be on program, right?"

"I eat pizza twice a week!" I agreed.

"The owners are really good, too. They like me and don't care if I order pizza or not. But it always happened as the time dragged on that I'd end up getting a second slice—I'd be having the mushroom and onion and I'd want to try another kind. And then I'd have something for dessert, some sweet pastry. And sometimes I'd also stop in for ice cream on the way back to school. And then I'd feel bad because it felt as if the decision was out of my hands. Every time there was a drill, I'd end up breaking down.

"But when we had a fire drill a few weeks ago, I finally was able to turn things around. At first I told myself, *Okay, I'll just have diet soda this time. I'll really stick to the program.* But then I kept thinking of something you'd said at the meeting—*You have to be honest with yourself, that's your number one job.* I'd already had my lunch—what was I doing heading for the pizza place? I must have stood on the street for fifteen minutes before I decided that it was just asking for trouble going back. Afterwards it seemed like a simple decision, but at the time I had to fight it out with myself."

"Yes, it's always that way," I agreed. "For me it was an important turning point when I started to be honest with myself. I never went the *I'll only drink diet soda* route, but I was just as bad. I'd always start out with a lie, like *I'll just have one.* But it would end up being one bagful. One pound. One box. One half gallon.

"But then I began to say to myself—*Why should this time be any different? I won't just have one!* I became more honest. I began to admit to myself that the whole world is not out there eating. I stopped telling myself *I'll get away with it.* A box of doughnuts always showed up in the past, so why shouldn't it now? When I refused to believe my own lies, things began to change—and that's what you're talking about."

"So what did you end up doing?" The Beauty Parlor Owner asked The Secretary.

"At first I thought I'd take a long walk," she answered, "but I just didn't feel like it. I've been doing my exercise on the weekends and that's enough for me. So instead I did some window-shopping in the neighborhood and then I went to the library, where I had a great time catching up on the reading I usually never have time for. In fact, I got so into it that I was almost late getting back to work."

"Do you see the breakthrough you made that week?" I asked her. "I think we should not only add it to the list, but put it at the top."

I won't say The School Secretary was any happier with her slow loss that week than she'd been in the past. But maybe our meeting helped her to see that her victory was just as important as a lower number on the scale: she'd put a stop to a self-destructive habit and replaced it with a good one. She won't be at the mercy of those school bells in the future, and it won't mean a weight gain for her every time they ring for a drill.

What I especially liked about her decision was that she did *not* feel compelled to spend the two hours exercising. Of course, it's true that if she'd gone for a long walk, she would have sped up her weight loss *that week*. Some people might have chosen to do that; they might have enjoyed a brisk walk as much as reading in the library. But *she knew herself,* she knew her limits, and she'd realized that for *her* it would have been too much to start exercising in the middle of a workday.

People who try to do too much too quickly usually end up sabotaging themselves. They start a routine and when they find themselves unable to keep it up—for whatever reason, either because it's too hard physically or psychologically—they give up completely. If The Secretary had pressured herself into exercising this time, the next time there's a drill, she would be in more danger of lapsing back into her old habits. The feeling—*No, today I just can't bring myself to go walking*—might take over and what would naturally follow from that is—*Then I might as well eat,* an attitude leading her right back to the pizza parlor. This is a pattern I've seen often.

But The Secretary resisted this temptation—and it *is* a temptation, the result of wanting to reach goal weight as soon as possible—so that *now* the next time there is a drill she will remember how much she enjoyed browsing and relaxing in the library. Plus, she will remember the guilt-free feeling afterwards, the pleasure of being in control and being closer to her goal if only by a half-pound. Instead of dreading a long walk she doesn't enjoy, now she can *look forward* to her free time as an unexpected bonus—and that is the basis of permanent change.

When you consider all this, doesn't it seem unimportant whether she lost a half-pound or three pounds that week? Yet until our discussion, it never occurred to her to value her victory the way it deserved to be valued. She practically took no notice of it and, in fact, if it hadn't been for her friend's mentioning it, she wouldn't have brought it up. I certainly had no inkling the week before. All she'd talked about then was the hysterical feeling we've all had at one time or another: *"Oh, my God! I've only lost a half-pound! I might as well eat, I might as well be "enjoying" myself if I'm not going to lose—I'm going straight from this meeting to a bakery and eat as much cake as I want."*

She had actually paid her weekly fee for the meeting with her credit card to have more cash on hand for her binge. *"I only stayed after I weighed in because I had to return an umbrella I'd borrowed from my friend and I thought I might as well wait inside. I didn't plan on sitting through the meeting to the end."* But during that meeting, she'd calmed down enough to give up her bingeing plans. All of which shows how easily we can cheat ourselves of the enjoyment of our own achievements.

Making the Scale Work For You

Keeping all this in mind, there's still a lot to be said for the scale. Over an extended period of time the scale is a useful way of charting your progress and it can even inspire you. I know a young man in his early twenties, I'll call him Learned A Lesson, who'd been having terrible back pain and his physical therapist told him that one of the keys to getting over his problem was to lose weight. During the course of about a year he managed to take off about fifty pounds and is committed to losing the remaining ten pounds. He told the group during one meeting: "When I first saw my PT he gave me some twenty-pound weights to hold and said, 'This is what you're carrying around every day, all day. This is the extra strain you're putting on your back'—and I never forgot that. When I go to work out in the gym, sometimes I pick up two twenty-pounders and think: *This is what I've taken off!* It keeps me in line."

When he handed him those weights, his therapist made him face what he was doing to himself. It was impossible to hide from the stark reality of the numbers. *Here,* he was saying to the young man, *These discs weigh sixty pounds. Period.* And that stayed with Learned A Lesson over the year he took off the weight. He made the numbers work for him, not only in terms of starting him off but also at the end of the year when he used the numbers to help him make his achievement concrete. *I have lost this much!* he could say with satisfaction, summing up a long period of effort and self-control.

The moment a person takes that first step onto the scale, they are signaling a willingness to face reality. Most people with a weight problem know on some level that their eating is out of control, but by not finding out the exact numbers, they're able to persuade themselves that there's no urgent problem, that taking action can wait.

There was a lawyer in her forties who never missed a meeting over a long period of time—and this though she was in a very responsible position, was obviously a busy woman, and chose to attend meetings in the middle of the day in Manhattan. Every Thursday afternoon I could count on her to be in her seat before I arrived (and I always arrive early). She once told me what made her so committed: "I realized that I had gotten my priorities all screwed up. You know how I got the way I am?" she said, patting her stomach (she had a long way to go). "I kept putting off thinking about my weight. I'd promise myself that I would *do something*— but at the same time, I'd tell myself that first I had to finish this project or that project.

"I lived from deal to deal. I remember once planning on going to Weight Watchers®—it was very convenient for me since my office was just a few blocks away. But then I had to fly to Hong Kong and I thought, *What am I going to do? Start dieting in a Hong Kong hotel?* After that, I was working my ass off to get things going on another important project—and things never go smoothly. From week to week different problems came up and when I left the office, my personal life wasn't easy, either. My father was sick and my mother needed all the help she could get. My kid needed someone to give him a talking-to. And at the end of the day I needed *something* to relax me, right? The idea of going to a meeting and weighing in seemed like just one more strain, and I couldn't take any more. There was no time to worry about how much I was gaining and anyway, I told myself, *Oh, I'll knock it off in a couple of weeks. I always do. A few pounds can't hurt me.*

"Somewhere in the back of my mind I was still eighteen and able to eat cheeseburgers and ice cream sodas and never put on a pound. But when I finally got onto the scale, I saw what I'd done to myself: I had fifty-five pounds to lose. It scared me enough to stop me in my tracks. From now on, *this* comes first. Because if I eat myself into the grave, what good is everything else I do?"

A smart woman! She had to learn a lesson that many people forget: *Just because you don't go on the scale doesn't mean the weight isn't there.* The longer you stay off the scale, the more damage it's possible for you to do. This woman needed the shot of reality that only the scale could give her. Subconsciously we think that if we don't see the number, we haven't really gained the weight.

Frequently, I've seen members who have been doing well suddenly stop coming. Sometimes they then reappear six months or a year later with all the weight back on. "I had a bad week," a woman I'll call It Just Happened That Way said. "I didn't know how much I'd gained and I didn't want to know. So I decided to skip a week and be very, very good so that when I came back two weeks later, whatever I'd gained would be off. I was afraid of my reaction if I had to go on the scale that week. But what happened was the second week, I broke down after a few days so that another week went by, and somehow I never ended up coming back. I never planned on quitting—it was just that I was having a hard time and after a few weeks I kind of gave up without realizing it."

But when you're having a hard time, that's when it's most important to attend the weekly meeting and get weighed in. It's a first step—and when you take one step, another follows and then another and before you know it, you're back in control.

Rosalie's Seven Commandments for Facing the Scale

Let me sum things up with what I call *Rosalie's Seven Commandments for Facing the Scale.* They are based on years and years of watching so much success or failure as a result of the numbers.

ONE: SEPARATE THE FEELINGS FROM THE NUMBERS

Hold on to the feelings you had before you stepped onto the scale, whatever it says.

If the number on the scale disappoints you, ask yourself *How did you feel before you got on the scale today?*

If you were excited and happy because you knew you had done well, then it's a crime to let the number bring you down.

TWO: USE WHAT YOU'VE EATEN, NOT THE NUMBERS ON THE SCALE, AS YOUR GUIDE

If you lose weight, review the week and ask yourself: *What did I do to make this weight loss happen?* Be specific so you can remember what you've done for the future.

If you've gained weight, be honest with yourself. If you know you've done well, *forget it and go on to another good week.*

If you think about it and realize that you need to tighten up your control, then decide: *What do I want to change? How do I change it? What behavior or situations contributed to my not doing well this week?*

THREE: BE REALISTIC

If you're unhappy about the amount you lost (or didn't lose), consider your age, sex, size, your overall weight-loss rate, and then ask yourself: *What is a realistic expectation?* Don't compare yourself to others or even to yourself as you used to be.

FOUR: WEIGH IN EVEN WHEN YOU'RE GAINING WEIGHT TO HELP STOP FUTURE GAINS

Remember, whether or not you know the number, it's *there.*

FIVE: WEIGH IN ONCE A WEEK

You can do a lot of damage if you wait longer than this.

SIX: KEEP YOUR EYE ON LONG-TERM SUCCESS

Remember the number you started at—and look at where you are now! See the total picture.

SEVEN: REFOCUS FROM THE NUMBERS ON THE SCALE TO YOUR BEHAVIOR

Always keep non-scale successes in mind: they will help to overcome disappointments.

*   *   *

Most important, REMEMBER: We can discourage ourselves, we can weaken our motivation, we can lay the groundwork for disaster—OR we can encourage ourselves! We can strengthen our motivation and lay the groundwork for success! The scale is not my friend and it's not my enemy. I'm my own best friend or my own worst enemy. It's up to me what I'm going to be.

CHAPTER EIGHT

The Holidays—A Survival Kit

"What the holidays bring you depends largely on what *you* bring to the holidays."

—Rosalie Kaufman, Group Leader

Let me begin by saying that nobody ever got fat on a holiday. You don't put on forty pounds in a day or even in a week. So why the hysteria when I announce to the group: *Ladies and gents, the pilgrims are about to land again?* Why the groans, the sighs, the pained laughter?

There's so much tension in the air as the holidays approach— so much fear and anxiety that you can literally feel it as you walk into a meeting. Everybody has at least one *I remember how much I gained last year* story. Everybody has a major challenge facing them. Everybody is worried—*How much will I put on this year?*

One woman in my group offered her explanation. She has been a member for quite a while and is a very attractive woman in her mid-thirties who dresses with flair and who has worked so hard at losing twenty pounds that I feel as if I've lost those pounds with her. I'll call her The Hard Worker.

"I don't look forward to Thanksgiving, to Easter—Christmas is the worst," she said the minute the subject came up. "For me the holidays jeopardize my control. They throw me off my routines. They destroy everything I've worked so hard to achieve. And what you say about them only lasting a weekend or a week just isn't true for me. I start eating even before the holidays have begun— they've almost started, so what the hell? Or I eat afterwards, telling myself I've gone off it already, so I might as well keep enjoying myself. I've had years when I was still celebrating Christmas in August."

"Okay—so what you're saying is that you get demoralized during the holidays and that knocks you out for a long time," I replied.

"Yes," she nodded and there were other heads nodding around the room—the majority, in fact. "Any suggestions?"

"Yeah, spend Christmas at the North Pole!" a very sweet woman, an accountant who'd lost thirty pounds, called out.

"Maybe you should start by asking yourself why you get so demoralized," I suggested.

"That's easy," The Hard Worker answered. "It's because I gain weight every damn holiday."

"Let's try an experiment," I said. "How many people in this room can live with not losing weight this Christmas or Hanukkah? How many of us would be happy just to stay the same?"

Around thirty hands went up.

"Now, how many people here would say that a one- to two-pound gain is realistic for them?"

About twenty-three of the thirty people raised their hands.

"How many could put up with a five-pound gain?"

The remaining hands went up—with the exception of The Hard Worker.

"I want to keep losing," she said with determination.

"All right—if you want it that way, it can be done. You have to make up your mind and be very focused."

The truth is that it doesn't matter whether you've decided to lose, to maintain, or to gain a fixed amount of weight. What's important is to *remain in control*. To set an upper limit to how much you're willing to gain.

This goal often depends upon your rate of weight loss. On the one hand, if you lose three or four pounds a week, then a five- or six-pound gain is no tragedy. On the other hand, if you lose a half pound a week, those same five or six pounds become a disaster. In deciding this goal it's also very important to think back to other holidays: What were the challenges? Were they a difficult time, and if so, would extra food help you get through them? How much extra food? The more cautious you are, the more realistic your plan will be—and the greater your chance for success which is spelled CONTROL. Control must be your number one goal. What does it matter if you lose weight during the holidays, only to go out of control afterwards? Remember, being in control is not a numbers game but a term change of your life patterns.

When people first start out and they're very motivated, they often lose weight during the holidays. At the time, the desire to be thin *outweighs* everything. But when they've been on track a long time and motivation is low and temptations are great, then the desire to eat balances the desire to lose weight. That's when you are in danger of losing motivation and gaining an awful lot. I think of it as an old fashioned balancing scale: the desire to be thin is on one side, the desire to eat more is on the other.

"Just remember," I told The Hard Worker, "there's nothing wrong with deciding to give yourself some leeway. You become demoralized when you're too hard on yourself, when you set yourself goals that are unrealistic given where you are and the way you feel *now*. And when you can't live up to those goals, that's when the *What the hell* attitude takes over and you're in trouble. When there's a huge gap between what you expect and what really happens, it's easy to become discouraged and give up."

I'm sure she tried her best, but that particular holiday season she gained weight. She broke down in the middle of the week at a party they were giving at the bowling alley where she worked. She had some cake which, actually, fit very nicely into her program. But she panicked: she didn't stop to think, and on the way out of the bowling alley she decided to stop at a Carvel's in the neighborhood—an old hunting ground—and have the ice cream that she used to eat by the quart. And so it went for two days until she was able to get back on program.

In my opinion, her real challenge, ironically enough, was the weigh-in, not the holiday. She'd gained four pounds, and *now* she had to ask herself, *What next?* Actually, that question was made much easier because she didn't have to ask it alone, facing her bathroom scale, with a table covered with Christmas party leftovers in the next room. She was asking it on a freezing cold morning when she'd gotten up early, gotten dressed, and come out to a meeting. Furthermore, in the next room was a group of committed people struggling with the same problem. *Show me what a person wants, and I'll show you who that person is,* the Russian playwright Chekhov said. Coming to the meeting showed that she wanted to change, and the desire to change is *already* a change for the better. She wasn't content to wallow in her misery or to pretend that nothing was wrong, that this is the way she wanted things to be.

So it turned out that what was *next* for her was *going back on program,* and that decision was more important than any weight she'd gained or lost. She'd broken a pattern—the overeating had been isolated to two days at the end of the holiday week—and now she had a new pattern to live up to in the next year.

For her, going to the meeting was the renewal of the struggle, a sign of her renewed commitment; for others it might be a long walk, buying vegetables, returning to any of the routines we've put in place to support our new life-style. The point is that once the effort is made—whatever effort that happens to be—you're heading in the right direction.

Of course The Hard Worker complained very bitterly about the holiday and about how unfair it all was—but that's what the meeting is there for.

"Four pounds! Four pounds!" she kept repeating. "I can't believe the scale can be so cruel!"

"I'm very glad to see you back this week," I said. *"Congratulations!"*

Although she was very upset, still she understood. She took a deep breath and even managed to smile.

One woman in another group of mine, a theatrical agent, is persistent and successful in her field, but she threw in the towel so easily when it came to weight. She had joined an early morning walking group, and dropped out after the holidays. "I gained seven pounds between Christmas and New Year's and felt I was back where I'd begun. All my hard work was down the drain. How many hours would I have to walk, how many gallons of water would I have to drink to lose those pounds? So I gave up."

Of course, she's not being logical—the weight is there anyway. What's done is done. Which is better, to keep on walking with her additional weight or to give up? Giving up will help those seven pounds turn into twenty like compound interest. But since when did logic have anything to do with it? The incentive is gone because the woman looks down at her middle and sees what she's done to herself again.

The key word here is: AGAIN! She's thinking about her failures. She's thinking about her past dieting efforts that ended in disaster! She gets discouraged and stops thinking of the future just when she should be hanging on for dear life to whatever routines she's established—good habits bring more good habits, and bad habits encourage worse ones.

"If you were trying to get a booking for one of your clients," I asked her after the meeting, "would you give up after one or two NOs? Of course not! Why don't you think of it that way?" I was trying to give her some food—for thought.

Special Holiday Challenges

The truth is that there is usually a little disappointment after the holidays. Those who gave themselves permission to gain one pound beforehand frequently gain two or three; those who would have been happy just maintaining often ended up putting on a pound or two.

But this kind of disappointment is bearable. It's important to remember that *compared with the major eating disasters of the past* they are successes, especially if you think of all the pressure people are under at this time. Because in America we don't have *a holiday*—we have a *holiday season*. It can start with the Halloween candy and end in the middle of January—or later. Nobody talks about *Thanksgiving Day*—they talk about *Thanksgiving Weekend*. It's not *Christmas Day,* it's *Christmas Week*. And even New Year's—no matter what day of the week it falls on, people arrange their work schedules to make it a holiday weekend.

Then, there are endless rounds of parties at work. People are anxious because of all the time spent shopping during the Christmas season—and because of all the money spent, as well. If it's not a gift holiday, they still spend money dressing up the kids. They also know that they themselves will be looked over by the family and friends.

If they're used to being on a tight schedule at work, just having all that free time, all that *unstructured* time can get them in trouble. If they are having guests, there's the added strain of preparing and making sure the house is in order. If they're going out, they have to adjust their eating to whatever is being served. They are seeing relatives they might not normally choose to see, either their own or those of their spouses. Most times, they don't stop and consider all the reasons they are feeling pressured or anxious. They just let that anxiety translate itself into *I WANT TO EAT.*

And even when families get together with a great deal of love and joy, the emotions stirred up at these reunions may lead to overeating. Your guard is down. You are caught up in the moment. You are not thinking, *Let's see, is that one bread or two I've just eaten? Is that two hundred calories—or four hundred?* You enjoy yourself. You let go—and that is perfectly natural, normal, and healthy. If only we could accept that and take the consequences in stride, there would be no problem. The problem comes when we get demoralized by *what is normal* and make it an excuse to extend our holiday eating all year round!

Nostalgia plays its part in all this, too. We want to recapture an earlier, more carefree time in our lives, to eat the same foods we ate when we were kids. It's as if the food is somehow magical: we take a bite of gingerbread—in my case, potato pancakes—and we're back in our mother's kitchen, being taken care of again. Added to this, there's the depression, the sadness which many people feel during the holidays which makes them turn to food, the great solace. The ghosts of all the past holidays haunt them.

A usually upbeat, very attractive woman who has, though, about forty pounds to take off (for her health as well as her appearance) said to me after the holidays, "We used to have these big family meals at my mother's home in Brooklyn every Christmas—we were three sisters and two brothers. I was the baby. My father died when I was young and my mother raised the family on her own and we all kept together pretty much until she died. But now it's not the same. My brothers aren't speaking to each other, one of my sisters moved away, and I'm divorced and living alone. When I go to my sister's house I can't help remembering the way it used to be and that makes me so sad that I just eat everything my mother used to make for us. I guess it's my way of remembering—I don't know what's wrong with me."

"*Nothing's* wrong with you!" I said. "You're a sensitive, feeling human being! So you needed the food this year—maybe by next year you'll have more control if you keep working at it. After all, with time and patience you can achieve anything you want to."

But I could see that she was skeptical.

"Look at me," I went on. "If anyone had told me twenty-two years ago that I would get on an exercise bike when I felt upset, I'd have told them they were out of their minds! But now, that's just what I do—sometimes."

"Sometimes?" she asked.

"Yes, sometimes," I answered. "There are still times when I turn to food, but not *every* time, the way it used to be. And that's how I've stayed thin. Sometimes I go to the theater, sometimes I take my grandchildren out shopping, sometimes I get on my exercise bike. Sometimes I eat a huge stir fry. And sometimes I binge! You had a hard time this Christmas—okay. You're back here now, and my money's on you." And I meant it. I could see that she was a very determined person with a lot of strength—and one of those strengths, although she didn't know it, was the fact that she was so in touch with her feelings. They may have overwhelmed her during the holiday, but in the long run, with the proper techniques, I'm sure she'll succeed.

It's not only memories and nostalgia that the holidays bring up, of course—there are darker emotions, darker feelings. We feel deprived, we begin to pity ourselves when we see what we will be missing: *Why can't we just eat like everybody else? Why can't we let ourselves go for once?*

Everything is magnified at this time of year: if people are lonely, they feel this way times ten during the holiday. If they are in mourning, the holidays heighten their grief. If they are going through a life crisis, the holidays bring that fact home. With all this going on, is it any wonder that the temptation to binge is stronger during this time? But I always ask: *Is there anyone sitting*

in this room who has a problem that gaining five or ten pounds
will make better? If you do, I'd like to hear it.

A woman going through a painful divorce said at a meeting
that took place after Thanksgiving: "We're not a very close family
but we always get together on Christmas and this was the first
time I was going without my husband. Even though nobody said
a word, I knew they were all watching to see how I'm doing—my
cousins, my aunts and uncles. I seriously considered staying home.
But I went—"

And ate—*smart woman,* no, make that *experienced woman!*—
a huge salad *before* she showed up at the gathering, bringing along
two plates of healthy foods as her contribution: a beet salad, a
huge plate of tropical, out-of-season fruits, star fruit, pineapple,
kumquats, strawberries, cherries, blueberries. (RULE: *NEVER*
SHOW UP AT THESE HOLIDAY GATHERINGS HUNGRY.)

The Ghost Of Holidays Past: Making Use Of Our Experience

One woman, I'll call her The Daughter-in-Law, said at a meeting
that took place *two* weeks before the holiday, "Every year I go to
my husband's family for Easter simply because they live nearby
and my family never made a big deal about Easter. It should
actually be a joyous time for me because it's when my first baby
was born, but over the years I've come to dread it. I know in advance
what's going to happen—there are no surprises. My mother-in-
law will get to me the way she has every Easter since I married
her darling boy. She'll pamper him and worry about him and give
me little digs."

"Oh, I used to have that when I was your age," a woman in
her seventies said, "but I put my sister-in-law in her place and
after that she never got out of line again. You can take it from
me, it felt very good."

"It's not so easy in my case," The Daughter-in-Law answered,
"because the kinds of things she says are hard to answer. They're
hard to pin down."

"For example?" somebody asked.

"For example—well, first let me explain that last Easter I'd brought over a huge aluminum foil roasting pan full of beautiful salad vegetables to make sure that there would be something for me there. This was something new for me. What I had done before was to eat so much—I'm embarrassed. I would have things that were high in calories and afterwards I would gorge on what my mother-in-law gave me to take home. So here I was, trying to do something good for myself by bringing over a lot of healthy food to make me feel satisfied—"

"To ward off a binge—" someone put in, and she nodded.

"I filled up my plate with vegetables, and while I was eating, my mother-in-law gave me a funny look and then looked over at my husband in a kind of worried way and said to him, 'Are *you* getting enough to eat?' putting a little spin on the word *you* so it's like she was saying to me: You *eat like a horse, but are you feeding him?*"

"He's a big boy now! He can feed himself," the older woman said and laughed.

"I know, believe me, I know. But a crack like that made me stop eating because when you're carrying as much weight as I am, it's hard to eat in front of people even though it was ninety percent vegetables made in a way I like them—with a little bit of oil, soy sauce, and low calorie dressing."

"Well, the question is, what are you going to do about it this Easter?" I said.

"I've been thinking about not going. I know my husband will make a big stink about it, but I just don't want to face it. Maybe I could pretend to be sick."

I could understand her feelings. Her mother-in-law's attitude toward her had stopped her in her tracks.

"Why don't you talk it out with your husband?" somebody suggested and she said she'd think it over. And that's what she did: during that week, she decided to trust her husband and tell him how she felt. But he was totally unsympathetic.

"He told me it was all in my mind," she said at the next meeting, "which I know is not true. So we got into a fight. I should have pretended to be sick and left it at that."

"You can't run away from things," an older woman said. "If you say you're sick this year, what are you going to do next year?"

"I'll be thin by then," The Daughter-in-Law answered.

"So? You'll still have the same problem," the older woman went on. "If your mother-in-law controls you, she can just come over or call and set you off. You have to deal with what's going on."

"Let's face it—you're using her as an excuse," a man said. "if I wanted to eat a stir fry instead of a chocolate cake, I wouldn't care about anyone. I could eat it naked in Macy's window."

"You'd probably enjoy that!" a woman called out.

Everyone laughed and then I said, "Think of how you can make this Easter different!"

"I don't know yet," The Daughter-in-Law said.

"Well, after all your months of coming here you know your options," I reminded her. "Just try to make sure you have a plan when you go to that gathering."

The holiday came and went and at our post-Easter meeting, she was the first to answer my question, "How did we do?"

"Great," she said with enthusiasm. "I stuck to my vegetables and nobody said anything. I guess they just got used to it. And when the killer came, chocolate mousse, I said to them, 'Don't wait for me—go ahead—I just need a breath of fresh air. I need to stretch my legs'—and I took a long walk by myself. I had planned it out ahead of time and I'd even left my walking shoes in the car—it had been a tossup between the walk and helping clean up the kitchen, but since it was such a beautiful day, I decided to get out. It was better than sitting around watching them eat. I had decided that that would really drive me crazy, so that's what I chose to make different this year."

"How did they react?" somebody asked.

"It was fine. My husband got some time alone with his mother, which made her nicer. I got some quiet time and some exercise. And when I came home, I went through my mother-in-law's care package, took out one treat for myself, and the next day sent the rest to my husband's office. Let him show off his mother's cooking, I decided after giving it much thought. I wanted to dump it then and there, but since my husband is so attached to his mother, I was afraid it would make him angry. But all that matters is that I got rid of it. That was the best part—I feel so good about myself now, I feel so strong."

I liked the creative way she turned a negative situation into a positive one—her "time out" walk was a way of doing something for herself, keeping to a healthy routine she'd gotten into *and*, I'm sure, decreased her stress so she was able to return to the gathering with more strength of will. Don't forget, these holiday meals are always late and then everyone ends up sitting around the table for hours and hours. There's pressure to conform: everybody's eating and everybody wants you to join in. What better way of breaking the almost hypnotic spell that food puts you under than a brisk walk?

I also liked what she said about taking out a treat for herself from her mother-in-law's care package—that part was just as important as getting the rest out of the house. There was no reason on earth for her to pass up everything—she could even have had the dessert with the others if she'd wanted it, but she chose to work things out her own way. First she had to prove to herself that she was in control by passing it up, and it worked for her *this time,* in this way. We must remain flexible and realize that next time, a different way might be better.

Let me stress the importance of what The Daughter-in-Law did when she took a treat out for herself—when she gave herself something. First of all, pure and simple, that was her way of saying to herself that she deserved something. Of rewarding herself, of standing up for herself. It was a good move and a good sign of how her self-image was changing.

Next, she prevented what is always a concern of mine—"delayed reaction." Very often, I find that it isn't always the day of the gathering that's the problem. Many people do well on the day of the holiday because they are so geared up for it that they deny themselves everything. They think they're very strong—and then they do a number on themselves the next day with food far less satisfying and interesting than anything they could have eaten on the holiday. During my years as a leader, so many people have told me how perfect they were on Thanksgiving Day—and how they ATE on Friday, Saturday, Sunday—up until the moment they came to the meeting.

In all my fat years I never allowed myself to eat. I never gave myself permission. I never said—*This is a holiday, it's okay to enjoy. It's okay to indulge a little bit; everyone has a right to eat a little of his favorite holiday food.*

I've said this before and I'll say it again since it's so important: *Every good weight loss program has to have room for an occasional indulgence, otherwise it doesn't work.* Only I never understood that, so I sneaked food on the side that I never thought I was entitled to eat. I never ate at the holiday table—so I ate while I was cleaning up, and then the portion I allowed myself was a big one: *Everything.* Everything left over. Everything I had wanted but had been afraid to eat publicly. Before I was married, I sneaked food so as not to eat in front of my parents, who used to give me a hard time about my weight. Then I'd sneak food so I wouldn't eat in front of my husband *who never cared what I ate.* I couldn't eat in front of him—but that was *my* problem because he didn't care what *he* ate, never mind what I ate. So who was I really sneaking away from? Myself?

The habit of never eating in public took over. Now I do the opposite; I keep no junk in the house, I *only* eat in public—and *in public* is a very controlled situation. One of the suggestions I would make to people who ask, *How do you eat a favorite food without loss of control?* is to eat it publicly. I thought like a fat person, so I remained one for a long time.

And it's not just about eating at the holiday table. It relates to a whole range of activities, from the way we dress to the way we stand. The *fat person mentality* takes over. Sometimes we don't go swimming or go to the beach in the summer because we don't want to wear a bathing suit. We don't eat with others because we feel they are judging us: people think that instead of eating, we should be living off our residuals. We don't dress in a stylish way— we don't want to call attention to ourselves so we hide in sacks. The Daughter-in-Law kept a treat for herself, for later, for after she was safely home. Maybe next year she won't have to do that— but what matters is that she felt good enough about herself to allow herself that one sample of what was good at the holiday table.

Strategies and Game Plans

Let's talk about what we need to bring us through the holidays. First of all, how about starting out with a little enthusiasm instead of dread? How about forgetting *I'm not going to eat the dessert,* and try saying: *I'm going to* have a great time! I'm going to enjoy the healthy foods I've brought along with me, including a fabulous low calorie dessert—OR—I'll have just enough of the traditional foods to make me feel satisfied—and no more!

Change gears. Why not resolve to help at least one other person have a better time this holiday—find at least one way to give of yourself during the family gathering? It'll help put the food urges on the back burner. I won't say it'll kill your sweet tooth—it won't. But you might end up enjoying yourself more.

For example, a lifetime member tells of a cousin who has a large family. One of the middle boys, a child of eleven, never gets enough attention—you can see he's a needy kid. Over the years, she has singled him out by telling him a story or playing a game with him or bringing him a special treat. She has become his favorite—when she shows up at a family party and sees his eyes light up, it gives her a tremendous lift. "I won't say it deadens my appetite," she told the group. "That wouldn't be true. It's a different kind of gratification, but still it's one of many ways I get through the holiday."

And let me tell you, young mothers are grateful if someone takes the kids for a while. If you decide to go out for a walk with a few of the little ones, everyone will bless you. Sometimes it's the elderly who could use a little extra attention. One woman who tried this method said, "My mother's sister is the kind of woman who if you say to her, *How are you?* she's good for a half hour. She loves to talk and ever since she's become a widow, she's been very lonely. Her own kids don't have the patience for her anymore, so I made a point of sitting next to her at the last family gathering. It wasn't fascinating conversation—but it made me feel good about myself and it distracted me from a table that was so full of rich desserts, you would have needed a computer to figure out some of the calorie counts." She'd discovered the principle which Mark Twain puts so well: *If you want to be cheered up, try cheering up others.*

Then we need the practical skills that can make a big difference. Knowledge of the food lists, important all year round, becomes crucial during this time since it helps you figure out how to work holiday foods into your plan—the *must-have* foods, foods you would feel cheated if you didn't have. Another skill is learning ways to make traditional recipes with less fattening ingredients— some members have become so skillful at this that their families actually begin to prefer the lighter, less fattening versions of old favorites.

Then there's what I call PUTTING AN END TO IT. Not letting the leftovers ruin us. Give those treats to guests to take home, give the food to the homeless, feed it to the pigeons if you can't bring yourself to throw it out—but don't leave it in the fridge or on the kitchen counter. It's a binge waiting to happen. We all know the, *Well, it's left over so I may as well as . . .*

A woman I'll call Feeling Desperate came up to me after the meeting and said, "It's when the holidays are over that I eat." She is a widow in her mid-forties who put on about thirty-five pounds after her husband died of cancer.

"When my parents got divorced I started putting on weight— I was just a girl then. But I've never been this heavy in my life," she said the first time she showed up at the meetings in the beginning of December—a difficult time to start.

"Don't focus on the problem," I told her. "Focus on the solution. You're overweight—so what are you going to do about it? Tell me one positive step you are planning to take!"

"I'm not going to gain weight this Christmas," she said and everyone applauded.

"Great," I said. "By joining now, you'll have time to work out a holiday strategy."

She did very well throughout Christmas week, but after New Year's, when her married daughter, who'd been visiting, went back to Arizona, she felt depressed. "The house had been full of guests and friends during the holiday—not only mine, but my daughter's. So after she left, I felt so lonely that I ended up eating. I could kick myself—I'd been so careful when all the temptation was around, and then I went out for no good reason and bought bagels and cream cheese and cake and ruined everything."

"But you *did* have a reason," I said. "It's hard after people you love go away. Especially when you're living alone, the way you are now. You tackled the holiday itself this year—next year you'll be on guard for the aftereffects. It's a slow process—but you've begun. Instead of focusing on the bagels and cake, why not congratulate yourself on what you've done well?"

The trick is to keep improving our habits and one way to do this is to learn from our past mistakes. As Thomas Edison said after going through over a thousand different materials he was testing to make the filament in the light bulb, *Well, now we know what DOESN'T work.* Valuable information. Think back to past holidays and use them the way you would a natural resource. They can help you avoid mistakes when you plan for the future and give you a sense of what you're up against now.

This is especially helpful when it comes to readjusting *emotional* expectations which can be just as important as setting realistic weight goals. Think of them as "emotional goals". At certain times of the year on Christmas or a birthday or other holiday, we think we should love each other. It's part of the holiday spirit—but people who don't get along all year, don't suddenly change because it's Christmas or Hanukkah. We bring all of our fractured emotions and stresses to the gathering and we have to learn to accept this fact, to make peace with it, as a way of coming through the holidays in a better frame of mind.

One woman in her fifties told me a story that underlines this. For many years she came to my Sunday meeting regularly—Sunday is her day for body and soul, that's her slogan. First Weight Watchers®, then church. When she dies and they lay her out in the box, she always says, her one wish is to be in her size ten dress, label out to show everyone. An intelligent woman—she works as an executive in a large department store—and a problem solver, the one problem she can't solve is the holidays: they throw her every year. As a young girl in her teens, she'd married into an Italian

Catholic family. But she saw that even though she became a Catholic, it was never the same as far as her husband's family was concerned. She felt that she wasn't really accepted the way the Italian daughters-in-law were; she was different; they were always looking to criticize her, and that would make her eat.

One year she came back to the meeting after Christmas and said, "I did something wonderful for myself and I loved every minute of it."

I thought she was going to tell us about the homemade cannoli she'd eaten, her mother-in-law's specialty. Instead, she said, "For the first time ever I *didn't* eat the cannoli. It was the best present I could ever have given myself. I finally, finally asked myself: do I really want this or am I only eating it because I'm not happy now? And that's when I decided to pass it up and have my own dessert later on when I got home. There was no way I could ever think of bringing it into my mother-in-law's house—she'd get too insulted."

"What made the difference this time?" I asked her.

"Just before we went over to the in-laws', something clicked. I was sitting in the car, resenting them, and suddenly I said to myself: *They don't like me, they've never really liked me. And you know? It's their loss.* I think that not wanting anything from them at long last made all the difference. I just told myself it was enough. And that was that."

But what do we do about the *must-have* foods, the foods that make the holiday the holiday, the delicious, tempting desserts that come along only once or twice a year? On Christmas it might be that sinful eggnog and the homemade Christmas cookies. On Hanukkah it might be the potato pancakes. On *any* holiday when I make stuffing, that's it for me. I make stuffing once or twice a year and when I make it, I want some and I'm not going to do without it! No way! But I plan it, I allow myself to have it. I give myself permission.

But a word of caution: How much I eat very often depends on how tired I am, how hungry I am, the state of my emotions. Lesson: over the years, I've learned that picking at the stuffing that falls out of the bird and into the gravy is *not* a good idea. That's the time when I'm tired, I'm anxious, people are coming; the house has to look right. I used to eat every holiday meal twice. Once hot—when it came out of the oven—and once cold, after everyone left and I was cleaning up. I'm very vulnerable to that kind of eating, so I've learned to protect myself with rules. I only eat sitting down; I always try to eat with dignity.

We have to learn the difference between controlled overeating and orgy overeating. One is an emotional decision and the other is like getting drunk, a loss of consciousness. I have had many occasions when I decided I was willing to pay the price for food that was just too good to pass up. Or—maybe the most irresistible food of all—food that was offered in love.

Let me close this chapter with a beautiful story that redeems the holidays for me—almost.

After two years of going up and down, one of my members was finally on a winning streak. She'd hit her stride and had been losing steadily for more than six months. After giving the matter a lot of thought, she decided that she was *not going to let the Christmas holiday come between her and success this year*. "Rosalie, I made a vow and when I make up my mind I'm a very stubborn person as my husband's always telling me. I knew what was coming—my sister is an excellent pastry chef (she works for *La Vie*) and my father, the person she got it from, bakes cakes that are out of this world—"

"Are they overweight?" somebody asked hopefully.

"My sister could be a fashion model."

Groans came from around the room.

"I know how proud they are of their baking, so I planned in advance not only to taste, but to eat what they made. I wanted them to feel complimented and honored because they've been so good to me. So I worked very hard all week. I kept thinking of what you said, Rosalie: *the only place success comes before work is in the dictionary*. I put an extra twenty minutes onto my exercise routine and cut back on all my optional calories, figuring I'd be safe enough to eat anything my relatives dreamed up."

"Did they know you were dieting?"

"That's just the point. I showed up with all those optional calories to my credit—ready, willing, and able to eat. But they surprised me: they had made a fabulous, healthy meal and baked *the most delicious low calorie chocolate cake I'd ever tasted—for themselves as well as for me.* There was no reason to go off program and there was no way I could. Everything on the table was both delicious and healthy."

"And what did you do with all those extra calories?" a member asked.

"I chalked them up to the spirit of the holiday."

"Amen," I said. "Now tell us: What was the recipe for that delicious cake?"

"That's a state secret," she said, and so we ended the meeting on a note of mystery.

Let me leave you with one last thought. In the springtime, some of my members celebrate Easter, some celebrate Passover, and others just greet the spring without any formal religion. In each case, though, it is a time of rebirth and freedom, a reawakening to that which is best in life.

When we shake off our bondage to food, when we refuse to remain fat and depressed and miserable, we are re-creating ourselves—and we can make that spring happen whenever we choose. Instead of making the holidays a time when we repeat past mistakes, why not make them a time of hope and change for the better?

CHAPTER NINE

The Long Haul—
Maintenance

"There's no free lunch."
—Adam and Eve after consultation with the snake

I may not be the person I want to be;
I may not be the person I ought to be;
I may not be the person I can be
But praise God, I'm not the man I once was.
—Martin Luther King, Jr.

There's so much ooh-ing and aah-ing when you first lose your weight. When you go to a family reunion, a wedding, or a party after you've reached your goal weight—or just when you meet an old friend who hasn't seen you for a while—you become one of the Seven Wonders of the Ancient World. They stare and stare at you as if you were the Hanging Gardens of Babylon. You're the center of attraction. You get more attention than the bride at the wedding. You're IT.

A year goes by—and this is the way you are. This is YOU. The thrill is gone. People are used to you this way. *You're* used to you this way. So what keeps you going?

Habit. Make that—new habits?

Remembering what things were like in your fat days?

Better looks?

Medical consequences?

New healthy foods you've learned to like *(Yeah, eggplant is really going to replace ice cream, right?)*?

Old fattening foods you've learned to eat in moderation?

Pleasure in exercise?

New pleasures like buying beautiful clothes or spending time with your loved ones instead of being in a sugar stupor half the time?

A better sex life?

An even better sex life?

More self-understanding?

More self-respect?

Taking this book down from the shelf and reading it through again and again?

There's no simple answer because *forever* is a long time. If we were told we had to be coal miners for just one day, most of us could do it. All of us could chop rocks for a day. But if someone said, *You have to chop rocks for the rest of your life,* you'd lie down on the floor, overwhelmed. That's the problem with the fight against fat. It isn't ever over.

Of course, we can pretend to ourselves that's it's only for a day—we can (and should) tell ourselves *Let's take care of today and forever will take care of itself,* but sometimes that doesn't work after we've been on track day after day, month after month, year after year. We get discouraged.

Take the case of a Weight Watchers® group leader named Rosalie who's had fifty pounds off for twenty-two years—any resemblance between her and Yours Truly is purely accidental. What does *she* do when the feeding frenzy begins or even when she's in a bad mood? And I must say that when she's feeling down, the recipe on the fridge door for cheesecake—cottage cheesecake— does not stop her from dreaming of the real thing.

How do I go on, feeling that way? Sometimes I don't. I break down. I gain one, two, three, four pounds. There are different ways of maintaining: maintenance doesn't always mean being at the same number every day of your life. I used to maintain just trying to stay within the limits of the program all the time, maybe adding a little extra food now and then; but that doesn't always work for me anymore. Sometimes I have to allow myself a "bingette" as opposed to a binge. I will gain, but I always stay within a narrow range of gaining between two and four pounds, never more, and then I go back on track and take them off. Sometimes it's a stressful occasion, but it could be a joyous one as well. The last family affair I went to was a bar mitzvah. I loved the people. I was happy to be there. I looked good *and* the desserts were fabulous. I just felt like eating more than I usually do, maybe more than was even good for me—but that's where it ended. When I left the party, I went right back on program.

It's a matter of isolating those overeating episodes and limiting them to a short period of time. When I go even a fraction of a pound over the four-pound limit I've set for myself, that's *it*; I know I'm in trouble and I put on the brakes.

At those times, I watch everything that goes into my mouth, every bite. Sometimes it's a bite of cake, however, so I get on my exercise bike—I don't say I pedal—I get on it. I get off it again, have another bite, visualize another fraction over those four pounds. *Wait*, I say to myself, *what's happening here? The eating stops this minute.*

Why this minute?, I ask myself. *You've eaten all morning—the day is ruined anyway. Why not wait until tomorrow? Tomorrow morning is time enough to get back on program.*

No, the Voice of Experience answers. *I want to wake up already back on program. That always makes me feel better. No more eating this afternoon.*

I call my daughters. Pick up a mystery novel with a suspenseful plot. Go to the movies. Take a walk. Buy something luxurious. Come back—and you know what? I still want to eat. *Oh God*, I groan, *this is so frustrating.*

What? my husband asks, poking his head in from the study.

I tell him, Thank God, I lost a pound this week. I don't want to make my problem his, if I tell him, he doesn't know what to say anyway.

He shrugs and goes back to his books.

This is it. This is the end. I've kept fifty pounds off for twenty years! And look what's happening now, I tell myself. I look up at the clock. It's dinnertime—if it were later, I'd go to bed and I know I'd wake up feeling better the next morning. But it's not late enough for that, it's dinnertime.

Skip it, I tell myself, *you've eaten all day. You've munched and crunched your way through the morning and now you're going to sit down to dinner?*

Absolutely, the Voice of Experience answers. *There's no way I'd miss eating that large pot of cabbage soup and meatballs I made when I still had my sanity.* It tastes like sawdust, like something I won't mention—but I eat it. Thank God. I am back on my routine. On program. Wednesday night menu: Cabbage soup and meatballs. The bottom line is, the minute I eat that soup and those meatballs, my commitment is renewed.

No punishment. No looking back. The binge is over—I've avoided mistakes I would have made in the past. Maintenance does not mean having "arrived," and it doesn't mean perfection. It means making use of the lessons we've learned along the way to pull ourselves back from disaster.

Special Maintenance Challenges

The problem with maintenance is that we're constantly making little decisions: *What do I eat now? How many calories will I use up? If I eat it now, what do I do on the weekend?* If it were a one-time decision, it would be easy, of course. But maintenance is moment by moment, day by day. The thought process, the choices never stop. And it's frightening to see how easy it is to slip back into the old eating habits.

Even though I've kept off my weight for twenty-two years, I don't let that make me overconfident: that sense of danger is healthy for me. I never take my new lifestyle for granted. I had to work to achieve it, and I have to work to maintain it.

In my case, there are two principles that save me. The first is that *I've learned to ignore my negative, self-punishing voice.* Sometimes that voice tells me *All is over.* Sometimes (just as destructive) it tells me not to eat my regular dinner since I don't "deserve" it or since I must make up for what I've already eaten. Sometimes it just tells me to wait until tomorrow. But whenever I hear that voice, I know it has only led me to nonstop eating in the past and that I must use different strategies if I am to succeed.

The second principle I've learned is *when I feel like giving up,*

I must do whatever I can to take care of myself, to substitute healthy pleasure for the self-destructive one of eating.

But chances are that when I am needy or in trouble, I look for the easiest way to give myself a lift. Bingeing on cake and ice cream is easier than going to the theater or making a healthy meal. It's the path of least resistance. I can start eating in as much time as it takes to walk to the local bakery.

As time goes by, we tend not to work as hard as we did at the beginning. We don't put the effort into our food. Shopping and preparing a delicious, low-calorie meal takes *so* much time. We stop going for the long walk we made a priority in the beginning. One by one, we give up the self-nourishing activities that helped us lose the weight.

It's like the story about the three old men, seventy, eighty, and ninety years old, sitting on a park bench when a pretty young girl walks by. The seventy-year-old says, "If I were young again, I'd hug her all night." The eighty-year-old says, "If I were young again, I'd kiss her all night." The ninety-year-old says, "If I were young again—what was that nice thing we used to do?" When the motivation goes, we can't even remember all the "nice things" we used to do for ourselves. Sometimes this is simply the result of inertia, but sometimes new problems arise, or the old ones get worse, and then the first thing that goes is "us".

When people fail to maintain their weight loss it is often because they stop being important to themselves—they stop putting their own well-being first and let themselves become overwhelmed by worry and grief.

In one of my groups there's a real estate lady, a very brave divorcée with a long weight history who is in crisis right now. She's fighting to stay on maintenance but doesn't know whether she'll be able to. She had been overweight for years, both as a young girl (her parents promised her an expensive sports car if she'd lose weight in time for her graduation from college—she ended up driving a secondhand Ford) and during her marriage; at one point, though she'd managed to get down to goal weight, it hadn't lasted long:

"The first time around, I chose a maintenance weight that wasn't realistic. I achieved it—but I stayed at it for about five minutes and never really had the satisfaction of enjoying my success. After one week, I put on a pound and a half, the next week I gained two more, and after that it was back to business as usual. I was always straining and striving to get back down to a really small size which just wasn't *me*. I was influenced by the styles, the fashions—everything is made for very thin women. Just go to the store and take a look at the way the clothes are cut, the way they're designed. But I never felt good at that low weight—my hands were always freezing, I didn't have energy. If I had just been smart and chosen a weight goal toward the middle of my range, instead of at the bottom—I'm big boned—I would've had an easier time of it.''

This is a common reason people fail to maintain their goal weight—they choose a number that's unrealistic. Any number is achievable, but we're talking about being able to maintain it COMFORTABLY for a long period of time. Sometimes what gets in the way is an image of ourselves from a "golden stage" in our lives that we want to recapture—we remember how we looked in our youth or during a time when we were happy. But to return to that weight may not always be possible or desirable.

Another factor is where you're starting from. Somebody who is five-foot-three and weighs one hundred and eighty pounds might be very happy to go down to one hundred and forty-one, whereas somebody of roughly the same height and build starting out at one hundred and forty-five might be *comfortable* at a lower weight.

The number you choose also depends upon your age. As we become older, a higher number often becomes more acceptable—which was the case with our Real Estate Lady. At first, she couldn't come to terms with the fact that she was no longer eighteen and it was only after she'd put back the weight that she was ready to reassess her goal.

All right—she miscalculated. She regained her weight and became so demoralized that she kept gaining. In other words, she put her weight back on "plus." Then came a painful divorce and the job of rebuilding her life. "I was in a terrible depression right after I broke up with my husband," she told me before the meeting one day. "My pride was hurt, everything that mattered to me seemed to go out the window. I thought we had such a good marriage and then I found out he was involved with a woman in his office. I'd been so patient and loving and concerned for him when he said he had to work late. Just the thought of them carrying on like that made me crazy."

Her divorce devastated her; she ate nonstop and drifted from day to day, letting the house go, letting the bills go, letting herself go. Her whole identity, her entire sense of who she was, was invested in that marriage. I read something that caught my eye in *The Times* the other day—*Today's women care more about getting a mortgage than getting a man.* But when she—and I—were growing up, there was so much fear and pressure when it came to marrying off a daughter. You don't hear words like *spinster* or *old maid* anymore, but you used to hear them all the time. That was the way she was raised, the values of her generation, which makes her comeback even more impressive.

"The first step I took was to throw out a cake I'd just bought. What made me? I was listening to the radio and I heard something worthwhile that Jack Dempsey once said: *A champion is someone who picks himself up even when he can't*—and that inspired me to try again." An important part of *trying* was stopping the bingeing. It made her feel better about herself and the control she got from being on program affected the other areas of her life as well. She rejoined Weight Watchers®, where she lost forty-five pounds in about a year and a half, going on maintenance and staying at goal weight for almost two years.

So you'd think, especially after she'd been through all that, that nothing could throw her. She'd been through the mill, she'd come out on top and things were going smoothly—until something happened that sent her back to food. She found out accidentally that her daughter was gay and the knowledge filled her with guilt and self-doubt.

"She always told me she was going out with guys, Rosalie. She was always talking about this boyfriend or that one. I thought we were so close, but now I see that everything between us was based on lies and that really hurts. Do you know how long she's been hiding things from me?" She started to cry. "I've been eating ever since."

"Why don't you talk things out with her instead of eating yourself up alive?" I asked.

"I don't feel I have the right. It's not something she wanted me to know."

My job isn't to tell people what to do with their personal lives, but my guess is that sooner or later, the moment will come when they will talk things through. For the time being, though, it's easier for her to eat than to confront her fears about that moment. The only question is whether she'll stop herself soon or whether she'll be talking to her daughter with an extra fifty pounds on her from worry and guilt—from all those *Why didn't you trust me?* feelings.

This woman's first response is, understandably, to eat. It's an old, old habit, whereas her healthy routines, her healthy techniques are comparably new. The fact that she's eating now doesn't mean she has to continue. Just the fact that she came to the meeting is a sign that she hasn't given up everything. She had been inspired before; maybe something at the meeting will inspire her again. There's an old Chinese saying: *That the birds of worry and care fly over your head, this you cannot change; but that they build nests in your hair, this you can prevent.*

How can we put the wisdom of this Chinese saying into practice? *RULE: EVEN IF WE'RE BINGEING WE SHOULD HOLD ON TO OUR SURVIVAL TECHNIQUES*—such as exercise routines, drinking eight glasses of water, eating healthy foods, and so on. One woman said: "What keeps me going is that I've learned to rest *before* I get tired. I've learned to eat *before* I get hungry." And when she says *learned* she doesn't just mean that she knows it in some abstract way. It means that it's become an automatic part of her life. She lies down to take a nap at certain "danger" points in her day, no matter what.

In the face of problems, sometimes we give in and binge—okay! It happens. That's life. But if we hold on to whatever healthy habits we've developed, those habits become our salvation. Why is this? Because maintaining these habits helps us feel in control. And feeling in control gives us *self-respect*.

Breaking Out of the *There-You-Go-Again* Syndrome

A very wonderful woman in one of my groups, someone who has raised a great deal of money for AIDS research (her son died of AIDS) said to me after a year of being on maintenance: "It's not just that I'm eating candy, it's that I'm eating candy *again*— it's the *there-you-go-again* syndrome, the feeling that I haven't lived up to my own standards. My husband says to me, 'You'll never change. It's the same old you'."

But by keeping up a new, positive habit—in her case it's walking—she has *already* changed. And this is true across the board. You might temporarily lose control over what you eat, a problem might make you slip, but you *always* have control over the walking or the water-drinking or just the self-talk, not beating yourself up. And this helps you keep trusting yourself and your ability to change. As Helen Keller said: *Optimism is the faith that leads to achievement.*

I read a magazine article that talked about the effects of stress on various workers in a large company, and the finding was that the top executives suffered less from stress than other employees because they felt that they had some control over their lives. So there it is—the feeling of being out of control increases the stress, and stress leads to more eating. A vicious cycle.

Take the example of someone I'll call The Brooklyn Woman, who'd been maintaining her weight for about two years before she was fired from her job as a radio dispatcher in a car service. "After they let me go, I went straight to the bakery and bought a Black Forest cake and an apple pie. I started eating the chocolate cake in the car but the funny thing about it was that as I was driving, I noticed it was ten o'clock and I reached into the back for the bottled water I always have at that time, no matter what. So I was sitting there with these two cakes and I caught myself thinking, *What good is the water going to do? I'm not thirsty. I'm not on program anymore, so why should I bother with the damn water? I hate it, it makes me run to the bathroom a hundred times a day, it's a real pain, so why should I bother?*

So there she was, completely demoralized and using cake as a crutch again. If you'd run the film back to where she was a few years ago, you'd have to ask, *What's the difference between then and now?* You could say *the weight she'd taken off.* But if she kept on eating like that, those pounds would be back soon enough. It takes a long time to lose weight, but gaining weight happens pretty quickly. It's like a piece of knitting—you can unravel months of work in a short time. What was the use of all those months on program? The answer lies, I think, in her description of her feelings and thoughts at that moment:

"It seemed so stupid to be drinking water and eating cake at the same time," she said. "Then the thought hit me that I always drank my water. I guess you'd drilled it into me how important water is—"

"Yes," I nodded, for I always stress how important water is, both for general health and for weight loss. It's a natural diuretic. It gives a feeling of being full. It helps prevent constipation. It performs a thousand and one healthy functions. And we often eat when what we really want, if we stopped to think about it, is a drink. We often fail to distinguish between hunger and thirst.

"All the time I was working I made sure to drink," she went on. "I never missed my six glasses—I know they should be eight—no matter how crazy things got. And people are always in a hurry when they call a car service—they're always yelling and shouting and then a lot of the time they're not even there when the cars show up. If I didn't let anything stop me while I was working, why should I let *them* stop me now? I thought. It felt like I was beating them out by keeping up with the water, so I drank it as I finished up the cake—or I should say, as I *tried* to finish up the cake, because I guess my eyes were bigger than my stomach. Or maybe it was just that my stomach shrank over the two years I've been maintaining."

Habit became second nature and that water became a lifeline to her healthier self; it was her link to a time when she was in control of her food and, more generally, of her life. Any one of the healthy habits we develop during our struggle with weight is just as important as the number of pounds we lose.

We may gain weight back, we may break our routines for a

while, but once established, they are so much easier to re-establish. If you develop habits such as "tracking," keeping a written record of everything you eat, or portion control, figuring out the size or the amount of everything you eat, they will stand you in good stead throughout the rest of your life. Once you've discovered how good it feels to be motivated and on top of your eating, you will always remember that, no matter what lapses occur.

A woman once said to me before a meeting, "Rosalie! You've ruined me for life! I sat down to enjoy myself with an old-style binge, but as I was eating, I couldn't stop thinking—*This has a lot of oil, that has at least five hundred calories, that's a whole day's portion of bread.*"

"So did you stop eating?" a curious member asked.

"No, but I stopped enjoying it. I heard her voice in my head. I kept thinking about that person who's falling down the stairs, you know the example you give. Telling us to catch onto the banister and not throw ourselves down faster."

"Well, did the binge stop earlier than it would have?" the curious woman asked again.

"I don't think so. Not really."

"Then what's the good of thinking about it?"

That's an important question to answer. This woman became *conscious* of what she was doing to herself. She didn't just sit there eating handfuls of peanuts and pints of ice cream, promising herself to diet tomorrow. She knew just how much food she was eating and how long it would take to get it off—and she didn't just know it in her head, she knew it in her gut. She felt it. She'll remember that it was less pleasurable the next time she wants to binge, and that will help. And the next time she binges, or the time after that, I am sure it won't go on as long.

The point is that sometimes you don't see the results, you only *feel* them, the way this woman did when her out-of-control eating was "spoiled" by my voice. But that is a step on the way to control—in this case, long-term control.

It doesn't necessarily have to be something negative that can send you back to food—a promotion or a change of lifestyle for the better can do it. Or a marriage—part of loving is eating together: when you're single, you come home and it might do to have a salad and a tuna fish sandwich; when you're married, there's someone else who has to be considered.

What do you do when you're on your honeymoon and your husband orders a great meal? Do you sit there asking the waiter how much oil is in the salad dressing? Oh, please! When he orders dessert do you tell your new husband, *I can't have that!* I can't tell you how many times I've heard that weight gain started on the honeymoon. It's a very familiar story. The bride doesn't want to make waves; she eats along with the man, conveniently forgetting that he is a man, that he might be taller, larger, more active, or just able to eat larger portions and more sinful things. One woman lost all the weight from her first marriage in time to look great for her second one, but after sex she became ravenous—all she wanted to do was eat. "I ordered up room service on our first night together," she said, "and now look at me, fifty pounds later!"

It doesn't even have to be a husband—it can just be a roommate who affects your eating patterns. A young woman who lives in Manhattan doubled up with an old college friend to be able to afford an expensive apartment and she noticed that it became more and more difficult to stay in control. "I've known my roommate for years, but I never realized how much she ate—and she's thin," the young woman said during one of the meetings. "Somehow, we'd get into late night talks, which involved her going into the kitchen and making sandwiches. I kept away from the cake, but even getting into the regular habit of late night snacking—something I never did before—got me into trouble. I tried to make up for those snacks by cutting back on my regular breakfast, and that left me hungry and more vulnerable in the afternoon when I came to my lunch starving. I just have to remember that I can't eat the way my roommate does."

"Exactly!" I said. "Roommates, husbands, friends—what do they have to do with us when it comes to food?"

Sometimes, when the weight loss has taken a long time, a half pound here, a pound there, with many "plateaus," many weeks of staying the same, a person is ahead of the game: they have a sense of what maintenance is like even before they reach goal weight. A woman in one of my meetings took almost four years to lose forty pounds. When she was an overweight teenager, her mother had taken her by the hand to the pill doctor and she'd used pills ever since. Up until she'd joined Weight Watchers®, her pattern had been a quick weight loss followed by a quick regain. Her forty-pound loss was a major breakthrough because it was the first time she had ever lost weight without diet pills. All during the time she was losing, she was unwilling to give up her desserts, and so she traded what she wanted to eat for a slower weight loss, ten to twelve pounds a year. She's had those pounds off for a long time, five or six years now, and that very slow loss prepared her for maintenance by teaching her two of the most important lessons you need to learn for long-term success: *We must eat what satisfies us, balanced by what fills us up. We can eat what we want but not all at the same time and not all on the same day.*

Those four years had also been a lesson in patience. The payoff was that she didn't begin maintenance feeling starved and deprived and ready to make up for lost time by bingeing. She had acquired a realistic sense of what maintenance was all about.

Diamonds—and Maintenance—Are Forever: Developing the Right Attitude For Lasting Success

In the years before I became a Weight Watchers® group leader— when I was still pounds and pounds away from my goal—I remember envying the people on maintenance. Whenever I'd hear them complain I'd think to myself, *If only I had the weight off, I'd be so happy that there's no way I'd dream of bingeing again.* I just couldn't understand how they could complain about anything. And this kind of attitude makes it dangerous for people once they reach their goal weight. The feeling of *I've done it!* is a good one, but without the sobering awareness of a new struggle that's about to begin, it's easy to relax, to loosen up too much and fall back into old patterns. It's necessary to remind ourselves again and again that we're not on a diet, which lasts a finite length of time. We're trying to achieve a new pattern of eating which lasts forever.

For me, it was only after years went by that I realized the struggle *never* stops. Even when there is no crisis looming on the horizon, there are always countless small—and large—decisions I have to make at every turn of the road if I'm to remain thin. Courage comes in all shapes, all sizes—sometimes courage means just letting ourselves feel the way we feel without the instant sugar fix. Sometimes courage means forcing ourselves to speak up for our own needs, to become more assertive. Sometimes courage means facing the scale when we know we've binged, not denying that we're heading for trouble. No matter how long we've been maintaining, we have to remember that the craving to eat in the old way, the temptation to let ourselves go, is always there. There may be times when it eases up for awhile—but it can return one-two-three.

"There doesn't have to be any cosmic reason for me to eat," one woman who had been on maintenance for six months said. "A piece of cake can happen. I walk into my office, I see a Danish on my secretary's desk, and before she knows it, she has to choose between her job and that Danish."

"You mean her *life* and the Danish," another woman in the group chimed in.

That's as true for people who've been maintaining for years as for people who've just started out. The sense of taste remains keen—never underestimate sensory stimulation as a danger. As a woman in my Brooklyn meeting put it, "You walk down Kings Highway and what do you find? Delicious smells! Food! You go to Kings Plaza and what do you see? Food! You go home and what are your teenagers talking about? Food! You turn on the TV and what do the commercials show you? Not only food, but happy, thin people enjoying it."

"So what does that have to do with you?" I said. "First of all, thin people have their own ways of coping with occasional overeating. We see them eating a piece of cake, but we don't see them passing up dessert at the next meal. I'm always hearing stories about this one's daughter or that one's cousin who can eat anything, anything at all and never gain a pound. *Very nice,* I say, *I wish that person a long life free of problems.* But there's an old saying, *When you turn green with envy, you're ripe for trouble.* If you have a hundred dollars, do you go shopping at Bergdorf's for an evening dress? It's the same thing when choosing what you are

going to eat. Sure, I'd like to be fueling a huge Rolls-Royce, but I've come to learn that my body's system is like an efficient sports car when it comes to the size of portions, the number of desserts I can allow myself. I have to be careful in every way.

The bottom line is, I tell myself, what if I give in and eat—then what? I will gain weight. Will I be happy with added weight? Of course not, I'll be miserable. So I would have to start again, struggling not to binge, struggling to regain control. Only this time, I'd be struggling-and-fat whereas now I am struggling-and-thin. All I've gotten by giving in is weight. I have made the decision that if I'm going to struggle anyway, I want to struggle at my thin weight.

A woman I'll call Been Through Rough Waters told of having been placed in a religious orphanage after her mother died. "My sister and I were about eight and nine and our father felt it was too much for him to raise two young children alone. So we were different from everybody because we had someone who came to visit us on Sundays. We were never hungry, but the meals were always plain—healthy food with none of the treats little kids love. When I was sixteen, I guess my father figured we could manage on our own so he took us home. And that's when I got my introduction to eating. I began to binge on cake and ice cream and I kept right on. I tried every kind of diet you can name—I'd lose a few pounds and then gain them back again. I went up and down for years, but I never knew what it was to stay the same. So now that I've finished losing the weight, when I come in and weigh in and don't see the numbers go down on the scale anymore I feel very funny—"

"Do you feel afraid?" I asked her, having heard this kind of reaction many times before.

"Yes, I guess that's it. Also, disappointed—I know this sounds crazy—since I know I don't have any more weight to lose. But I feel disappointed every time I get off the scale."

Been Through Rough Waters is in her late thirties, so we're talking about a pattern of more than twenty years. This is more common than you'd imagine: many people are always what I call "on the way"—they're always on the way up or on the way down. Part of what's motivated them up to now is facing the scale every week and seeing a loss. That incentive is now taken away from them, and they panic because it's hard to give up anything that's been part of your life for a long time—even a destructive up-and-down pattern. When they don't lose weight, they stop trusting themselves. In the case of someone like Been Through Rough Waters, just knowing that many other people who reach goal weight have her fears reassured her. "Is it normal?" she asked me more than once and although I hate that word—recently I read an article titled "Normal Is Only A Setting On My Dryer," and that sums up how I feel about it—I did reassure her that many, many people have her fears when they reach goal. What she needs is some time on maintenance to gain confidence.

Reaching maintenance is a crucial turning point. Especially in the beginning, maintenance requires just as much focus and attention as the process of weight loss because people are always testing their limits. Yes, you eat more on maintenance but not all that much more. Just how much food is enough will vary from person to person, so that now a period of trial and error begins during which the natural tendency is to relax control, to become less careful. But the truth is that now more than ever it's so important to keep up all the routines you've been developing to lose weight—if you've been weighing and measuring your food, don't stop *now* of all times (the portions have a way of getting larger). If you've been keeping a record of what you've eaten, weighing in weekly, exercising, these routines will be your anchor while you give yourself more freedom in terms of what you eat. I encourage people who've been coming to the meetings to continue on a *weekly* basis (even though Weight Watchers® only requires them to weigh in once a month) because you can do a lot of damage in a month. Sometimes someone who's been on maintenance a long time will say, *Why should I keep going to meetings? This week you're talking about food planning—but I know that already! It's no news to me!*

Well, I tell them: *If you have to get dressed and take time out of a busy day and take a bus or a cab and rush up a flight of stairs to hear what you already know—you won't keep forgetting it!* We need to be reminded all the time. That's human nature. And having a regular, set time to review the principles that keep us thin is a good investment of one hour a week; you'll reap the rewards in health, energy, looks, control.

These are substantial rewards that people often overlook or take for granted, especially after they've been on maintenance for a while. All kinds of unrealistic expectations make people forget these important benefits—they lose the weight and expect Prince or Princess Charming to show up and when he or she doesn't, they turn to food. They're so busy being disappointed that they don't appreciate the so-called simple benefits their weight loss has given them. *If only* they could learn to think of their health before they lose it. *If only* they could appreciate what it means to be in control of what you eat rather than having the food control you.

At a meeting where one member was feeling very depressed because she felt she "just could not do it," I turned to four lifetime members in the room, one man and three women, all of whom had succeeded in maintaining for several years. I asked them for the secret of their success.

"Getting into the habit of throwing out leftovers or tempting food . . ." one began.

"Getting used to my water every day . . ." another said.

"I always make sure a binge stops on the same day . . ." a third answered, describing her new coping techniques.

"I never let myself get too hungry . . ."

Phrases like "getting used to" and "I always make sure" kept coming up as they talked. The common denominator was a good habit that had replaced a self-destructive one. Summing up the meeting, I quoted a saying I'd heard when I went to school and which is as true today as it was then. I think it gets to the essence of what maintenance is all about:

> *Watch your thoughts—they turn into your actions.*
> *Watch your actions—they turn into habits.*
> *Watch your habits—they turn into your character.*
> *And your character is your fate.*

CHAPTER TEN

Food For Thought

I've often said at my meetings that no one can imagine how much food it takes to keep me thin! I eat like a truck driver. But apart from quantity, certainly, I eat tasty and delicious food—not gourmet food, but food that's filling and enjoyable. I eat what I like, what satisfies me, at times of the day that are right for me balanced with what fills me. It's like putting together the pieces of a jigsaw puzzle to make it work.

Although I want to share a few of my favorite recipes with you, the specific ingredients don't matter as much as the principle behind them.

Note how simple it is to prepare delicious, nourishing food, meals you can make for the whole family. You wouldn't expect your guests to eat a baked potato and cottage cheese for dinner, and you don't have to, either. What you need is a pinch of imagination, a dash of preparation, and a great deal of commitment to a person who has been shortchanged for far too long: YOU!

Let's start with a few recipes to give you an idea of what you can eat and STILL REMAIN THIN—I'll give you my personal favorites! And please remember that I am a petite lady with grand-children and that maintenance is not kind to petite ladies with grandchildren. We are the last underprivileged minority who put on weight in the twinkling of an eye and have to work like the dickens to take it off. But then, as the saying goes, *Life is not about playing a good hand. It's about playing a bad hand well.*

In the following pages, I'm more interested in showing you the way I think about food than in giving you exact recipes or a possible "diet". My cooking is the result of common sense, a hectic schedule—there's no way I can cook every day—and the need for tasty, well-balanced meals to keep from sliding back into my old habits.

Mock Potato Soup

1 large head cauliflower, broken into florets	Salt, pepper, seasoning to taste
1 thick leek or one large Spanish onion	Bouillon to taste
	Water to cover

Cook all ingredients until vegetables are soft. Cool. Puree vegetables and return to liquid.

Unlimited portions. NOTE: When "unlimited portions" is indicated in the following, it means just that! You can eat all you want, in whatever amount, and not worry about gaining weight.

You have a creamy white broth. After two days in the refrigerator and depending upon how hungry you are, it can almost pass for potato soup. This soup is one of my favorite winter foods. I call it a "comfort food" because it helps when you feel you need something hot, something soothing, something to make you feel taken care of.

This soup is easily "dressed up"—sometimes I put one or two teaspoons of grated Parmesan cheese on top. Sometimes I put a measured amount of croutons into the soup, which can also be eaten with onion and garlic flavored flatbreads on the side.

Fruit Slush

Put ¾ cup plain nonfat yogurt into a blender.

Cut any fruit into small pieces and spread it out on a plastic plate. Freeze for about an hour. (Keep semi-frozen fruit in a plastic bag—this keeps the pieces from sticking together. I particularly love mangos for this recipe. Diced peaches, nectarines, or apricots are also wonderful.)

With one package of sweetener add the fruit to the yogurt.

Don't blend until pureed but leave chunks of frozen fruit in it.

It's the closest thing to soft-serve frozen yogurt that you're going to get. I love ice cream in any way, shape, or form. I'd love to eat it every day, all day. If I could climb into a bathtub full of ice cream, I'd be in heaven. By eating the fruit slush every day, I satisfy the need in a low-calorie, healthy way.

Food selection information:

1 fruit
1 milk

Those who are not Weight Watchers® members can calculate the calorie count by converting:

1 protein/milk = 70 calories
1 fat = 40 calories
1 bread = 80 calories
1 fruit = 60 calories

Vegetables are a "free" food (except for starchy vegetables like peas, corn, potatoes, water chestnuts, and winter squashes, which are a bread). Unlimited portions.

Mock Potato Salad

1 head cauliflower, steamed
  till tender and then cooled
Grated carrot
Diced celery (optional)
Thinly sliced red onion
Vinegar, sweetener, salt and
  pepper to taste
Measured tablespoons of

Weight Watchers® [or any
other brand] fat-free,
cholesterol-free mayonnaise
dressing at 10 calories per
tablespoon (depending on
how many calories you want
to use); I like my salad
creamy

It's hard to give exact proportions of seasoning because it depends on the amount of cauliflower used. If you have a favorite potato salad recipe, use it—only substitute cauliflower for potatoes.

I have learned over the years that almost any recipe that calls for potatoes can use cauliflower as a substitute. The Mock Potato Soup is an example; the Mock Potato Salad is another. See the following recipe for Cauliflower Kugel.

Cauliflower Kugel (Cauliflower Pudding)

4 cups steamed cauliflower, mashed and WELL DRAINED
2 cups chopped onion sautéed in cooking spray till golden
2 eggs

4 tbs. bread crumbs, matzo meal, or mashed potatoes
1 tsp. salt
Pepper to taste
2 tbs. reduced calorie margarine, melted

Preheat oven to 350°. Combine all ingredients, spray 8″ square pan, and pour in vegetable mixture. Bake for one hour, then turn off oven. Leave kugel in the oven until it cools. Makes 4 servings.

Selection information:

½ protein
⅓ bread
¾ fat

Imagine an 8-inch-square pan—and you can eat a quarter of it! That's a huge amount of food for when you're feeling ravenous or facing a lot of temptation. In the course of a long, hungry afternoon, I've been known to eat half the kugel. It's "cheap" food—you can eat a lot and still fit it into your eating program.

Cabbage Soup
～

A very versatile recipe.

2 cups diced raw cabbage
2 tbs. shredded carrots
6 oz. tomato sauce
½ cup water

1 tsp. apple cider vinegar
2 packages sweetener
2 prunes diced or 2 tbs. raisins

Combine all ingredients in a small pot and bring to a boil. Lower flame and simmer for 30 to 40 minutes till cabbage is soft. May need additional water. Makes 1 serving.

Selection information:

1 fruit

Delicious with ½ cup cooked rice, which adds one bread selection.

This is especially terrific for the winter when you want to eat something that's hot, sweet—but not dessert-sweet—that you can use to stretch out a meal. It's great as a one-pot meal with meatballs (see next recipe).

Meatballs

After the cabbage soup is cooked, drop small meatballs on top and simmer for 20 minutes.

3 oz. ground turkey   2 tbs. tomato sauce
1 tb. seasoned bread crumbs   Salt and garlic to taste

Combine all ingredients in a small bowl and form into small balls.

Selection information:

   2 proteins
  30 bonus calories

One of my favorite winter meals is the cabbage soup with the meatballs and the added rice.

Total selection information:

  2 proteins
  1 bread
  1 fruit
  30 bonus calories

A HELPFUL HINT: Buy grated cabbage—that saves you use of the food processor. Cook in advance, as it tastes even better reheated. The reason I love this meal so much is the combined sweet and sour flavors.

Turkey Noodle Stew

Another one-pot meal!

3 oz. ground turkey
1 cup string beans, cut into
  small pieces
½ cup tomato sauce

¾ cup water
1 bouillon cube—any flavor
¾ ounce raw noodles

Heat small saucepan and spray with nonstick cooking spray. Using knife and fork, break meat into small pieces and cook till it loses color. Add rest of ingredients and cook on very low flame, covered, till all liquid is absorbed (about 40 minutes). Makes 1 serving.

Selection information:

   2 proteins
   1 bread
  10 bonus calories

This is the low-fat version of a dish that many of us loved when we were young. Most children enjoy ground meat and noodle combinations. So do I. I use the string beans to bulk it up.

My "Shoveling" Foods

These are unlimited foods that I eat when everyone else is so stuffed that they can't eat another bite and all I can think is, *What do I eat next?*

Sweet and Sour Squash

2 Vidalia onions, diced
5 or 6 zucchini
2 8-oz. cans tomato sauce

2 packages sweetener
1 tsp. apple cider vinegar (or more, to taste)

Sauté onions in cooking spray until brown. Add other ingredients and cook on a low flame until zucchini is soft. Unlimited portions.

I freeze individual portions of this recipe. Sometimes when heating a portion, I add ½ cup of cooked rice. This adds a bread selection. If I want to make a meal out of the squash I add rice and a measured amount of leftover diced chicken. I have my hungry days when I just need to chew and swallow and it doesn't matter what I'm eating. Keeping myself very full can sometimes prevent a binge.

Vegetable Soup

Combine in a soup pot:

5 oz. each: broccoli, carrots, cauliflower	2 leeks (carefully washed, clean of sand)
1 large red pepper, diced	3 bouillon cubes
Fresh mushrooms—6 to 8 oz.	Seasoning to taste
1 stalk celery	Water to cover

Bring to boil, cook covered for ½ hour. Puree vegetables and return to liquid. Unlimited portions.

HINTS: If you like a crunchy soup, add frozen vegetables of your choice when you heat your portion. I cook *cauldrons* of this soup and freeze it in individual portions. I love it with ½ cup cooked couscous, which adds one bread selection. It's also excellent eaten with garlic flatbreads on the side.

Vegetable Medley

A gorgeous, colorful vegetable combination!

½ cup water
1 medium onion, diced
2 small tomatoes, diced
1 large red pepper, diced
1 small green squash, diced

½ lb. fresh mushrooms, sliced
3 stalks celery, diced
Salt and pepper to taste
Paprika
1 bouillon cube, any flavor

Sauté onion in Teflon pan. Keep spraying pan and stirring onion until it is caramelized (very brown). Scrape onion into saucepan, then add remaining vegetables. Sprinkle with salt, pepper, and paprika. Add water and bouillon. Cook until vegetables are tender, 30-45 minutes. Unlimited portions.

Noodle Pudding

1 egg
⅓ cup cottage cheese (nonfat)
1-2 packages artificial sweetener
½ tsp. vanilla extract
⅛ tsp. cinnamon

½ cup cooked noodles
¼ cup crushed pineapple, in its
  own juice
1 tsp. raisins

Using a blender or food processor, combine egg, cheese, sweetener, vanilla extract, and cinnamon. Pour the batter into a bowl. Mix in noodles, pineapple, and raisins. Spray 3" x 5" mini-loaf pan with no-stick cooking spray. Pour in butter. Bake at 350° till brown on top, 40-50 minutes.

Selection information:

  2 proteins
  1 bread
  1 fruit

Makes a terrific lunch. Easy to carry to work. Great eaten warm or cold. Very filling, especially when eaten after a salad. It'll make your fellow workers jealous, especially those with a sweet tooth.

Pineapple Cheesecake

We're talking sinful—without the sin!

⅓ cup nonfat cottage cheese
1 egg
1-2 packages artificial sweetener

½ tsp. vanilla extract
½ cup crushed pineapple, in its
  own juice

Using blender or food processor, combine egg, cheese, sweetener, and vanilla extract. Spray 3" x 5" mini-loaf pan with no-stick cooking spray. Pour in batter. Mix crushed pineapple into batter. Bake at 350° till brown on top, 40-50 minutes. Refrigerate. Eat cold.

Selection information:

2 protein
1 fruit

Believe it or not, this is a cheesecake where you can eat the WHOLE THING! I usually have soup or a salad to start the meal and the cheesecake becomes the dessert, which I enjoy with a cup or two of decaf.

My Favorite Stir Fry

A huge meal!

3 oz. chicken breast in strips	SAUCE:
1 small onion, diced	1 bouillon cube, any flavor,
2 cloves garlic, minced	dissolved in ½ cup boiling
1 tsp. oil	water
12 oz. frozen stir-fry vegetables	2 tsp. soy sauce
1 cup cooked pasta	1 tsp. cornstarch
¼ tsp. salt	

Spray Teflon pan with nonstick cooking spray. Heat pan, then add oil and sauté chicken strips. Remove from pan. Add onion and garlic, sauté till brown. Return chicken to frying pan. Add vegetables and salt. Add soy sauce to dissolved bouillon, then slowly add cornstarch, stirring constantly so it doesn't lump. Pour sauce over vegetables and chicken in frying pan and add pasta. Cook covered 5-10 minutes. Makes one serving.

Selection information:

    2 protein
    2 bread
    1 fat
   20 bonus calories

This is a meal for a cold winter night when you need two dinners. I usually eat half, wait a while, and go back for the other half an hour or two later.

Apple Raisin Muffins

This is not an easy recipe but it's really worth the effort. WARNING: *Don't use liquid milk; be sure to use milk powder.*

Process in food processor or blend:

4 eggs	1 tsp. vanilla extract
4 slices raisin bread	½ tsp. cinnamon
6 packages artificial sweetener	When the batter is smooth,
2 tbs. reduced calorie margarine	pulse in:
4 tsp. baking powder	12 oz. apple

In large mixing bowl combine 1⅓ cups skim milk *powder,* the batter from food processor, and mix thoroughly. Spray a 12-muffin tin with nonstick cooking spray and divide batter equally and sprinkle 2 tbs. raisins over the muffins. Bake at 350° for 15 to 20 minutes till toothpick inserted into center of muffin comes out dry. Makes 4 servings.

Selection information:

1 protein
1 bread
1 milk
1 fruit
¾ fat or 30 bonus calories

This has been my favorite Saturday morning breakfast for twenty years. I take these muffins with me whenever I travel. They are great on an airplane or as a meal or snack while touring.

Blueberry Soup

I have had raves about this one! When you need a pick-me-up that's absolutely delicious—this will fill the bill! It's terrific as an entrée at the start of a summer meal or for an unusual dessert. It satisfies the sweet tooth while only "using up" a portion or two of fruit. It's smooth and liquidy but the fruit gives it substance so it's satisfying.

4 cups blueberries	1 package Sugar Free Raspberry
1 package sweetener	Gelatin
Water to cover	

Put blueberries and sweetener into a saucepan. Cover with water. Bring to boil, lower the flame, cover, and cook for about 20 minutes. Slowly add gelatin, stirring constantly so it doesn't lump. Cook five minutes more. Chill.

OPTIONAL: Serve with a few dollops of plain, unflavored yogurt to give it a marbleized effect.

I buy many boxes of blueberries, clean them, and freeze them in plastic bags when the price is lowest during the summer so that this dish becomes a year-round treat. I suppose one could buy frozen blueberries, but these taste better.

Bean Salad

1 lb. string beans, cooked	¼ to ⅓ cup apple cider vinegar
4-oz. can sliced mushrooms	½ tsp. salt
½ cup canned corn kernels	2 tbs. oil
½ small red pepper in strips	2 packages sweetener
½ small yellow pepper in strips	

Mix all ingredients and chill. Makes 8 servings.

Selection information:

¾ fat
10 bonus calories

This is a beautiful accompaniment to a fish or meat meal. It's colorful and it's got a zippy taste.

Imitation BLT
(Bacon, Lettuce, and Tomato Sandwich)

1 small pita bread
2 tsp. reduced calorie
  mayonnaise

lettuce and sliced tomatoes
1 tsp. Bacos

Cut pita in half and spread 1 tsp. reduced calorie mayo on each half. Pile on the vegetables, then sprinkle on the Bacos.

Selection information:

  1 bread
  1 fat
  10 bonus calories

This is a great "cheap" snack. If you're going out in the evening and want to eat light during the day—by "light" I mean not using up too much of your food allotment—this is the lunch for you! It's a sandwich without protein.

Tuna Cakes

6 oz. drained, canned tuna, flaked
12 oz. saltine crackers made into crumbs
1 egg, beaten

¼ cup skim milk
1 tbs. minced onion
¼ tsp. Worcestershire sauce
Dash pepper

In medium bowl, combine all ingredients. Shape into 6 patties, then broil on both sides till brown. Makes 2 servings.

Selection information:

   2 protein
   1 bread
   10 bonus calories

This recipe came from a member 20 years ago and I have been enjoying it ever since. In the original recipe, the tuna cakes were fried. This is the low-fat version. The saltine crackers give it a different twist.

Beet Salad

1 15-oz. can sliced beets, diced	1 package sweetener
	1-2 tsp. vinegar or lemon juice

Mix all ingredients. Refrigerate. (Unlimited)

Great as a side dish or snack. I like to eat half of this recipe mixed with ⅓ cup of plain nonfat yogurt (40 bonus calories) and diced scallions and cucumbers (NOTE: Put the scallions and cukes in at the last minute so they don't get limp). I got the idea from an article on cold summer salads written by Pierre Franey in *The New York Times*. His recipe called for fresh beets, boiled, peeled, cooled, and sliced. So I bought a can of sliced beets and diced them—I knew I could never go to the kind of trouble Mr. Franey recommended. Besides, I didn't want to get my hands stained purple.

Generally speaking, people who have been so careless about their eating habits or so pressured for time that they live on junk food have to learn to use their common sense and modify gourmet recipes to make them "do-able".

Picture how pretty the beets are when served over kale or any green lettuce!

Broccoli Soufflé

20 oz. frozen chopped broccoli, squeezed out, or 1 large bunch fresh broccoli

6 eggs, separated, at room temperature

1 large chopped onion

1 lb. zucchini, coarsely chopped

½ cup Weight Watchers® margarine or ¼ cup regular margarine

4 tbs. matzoh meal, bread crumbs, or mashed potatoes

1½ tsp. salt

Pepper

Preheat oven to 350°. Cook broccoli. Drain well. Process all ingredients except zucchini and egg whites in food processor until smooth.

It might take 2 batches so that the batter doesn't overflow. Pour batter into a bowl, add chopped zucchini. Beat egg whites stiff and fold into vegetable mixture. Bake for 1 hour or until well browned. Makes 12 servings.

Selection information (per serving):

½ protein
1 fat
10 bonus calories

This is great company food—it looks beautiful and can be prepared in advance (it is not a true soufflé that can fall flat). It can be served at the Passover Seder or at any holiday meal and is also a great favorite with people who don't have to watch their weight.

A Simple Idea—
Welcome to My Kitchen

Once every two or three weeks I make a huge pasta salad which becomes the base *for different meals:*

12 oz. tri-colored pasta	1 head broccoli florets
Approx. 8 oz. olives, sliced	1 small head cauliflower
1 red onion, slivered	Shredded carrots

Steam the broccoli and cauliflower. Cook the pasta according to package directions. Combine pasta, steamed vegetables, shredded onion, sliced olives, shredded carrots. Pour 12 ounces of fat-free Italian dressing over all. Stir to combine and refrigerate. Keeps for about two weeks.

Use a measured amount of pasta salad as a base. For example, a cup and a quarter of pasta salad equals two bread selections. (I allow for the vegetables, which are "free".)

What I mean when I say a "base" is that I'll mix a measured amount of pasta salad with tuna fish or cold, leftover chicken. Or I could use the pasta salad as a side dish. It's great company food— colorful and elegant-looking, if presented properly. The advantage is that I have the food already prepared. Bulk comes from the vegetables, energy from the pasta. The onions, olives, and dressing give it a zing! And look how little time you need. It's a great food for anyone feeding a family. Just think: The old you opened the fridge and found fried chicken or cake—more pounds to weigh you down. The new you has a healthy meal waiting. There may be some people, however, for whom pasta is a red light food and who would eat the two weeks' supply in one sitting. In that case, until such time as they have developed enough control, they should only prepare as much as they need for one meal.

Planning—Self-Knowledge—Flexibility

I try to strategize, to save my main meal for when the need is greatest. For some people that might be in the evening—a lot of group members tell me they like to unwind after a hard day by eating a large meal and then snacking throughout the night. They eat a light breakfast and lunch and "save up" for this luxury. Others need a lift in the middle of the day or else they're lost.

Everybody's different—the trick is to get to know your needs well and then plan. That's the key here: *PLANNING, SELF-KNOWLEDGE, and FLEXIBILITY!* If I mention my case, it's just to give an idea of what I mean by a *strategy* to get you through the day. You'll have to come up with your own, depending on your needs. That means taking careful note of how you feel at different times of the day and trying to discover your pattern. It's also a good idea to see whether there's any special time during the day that you're more susceptible to bingeing. Think back over past out-of-control eating episodes. Did they take place regularly at any particular time? If so, be ready with extra comfort food or low-calorie desserts!

I'm ravenous in the morning, but I also need food at regular intervals during the rest of the day. I like a breakfast that consists of a bread, a fruit, a milk, and a protein. I'll mix blueberries with cottage cheese, for example, or have yogurt and flatbreads. Sometimes I leave out the protein and double up on the bread—a cup of hot cereal and fruit. I don't eat everything in one sitting. Before I exercise in the morning, I might take coffee with half of a bread serving. When I come back to the kitchen an hour later, I'll have the next part of the breakfast, which could be the fruit and cheese or an egg white omelette with sautéed vegetables, the vegetables having been prepared the day before including mushrooms, onions, and peppers to bulk it up.

Given my routines, there's no time in the morning to start sautéing vegetables, so I always have a few days' supply ready to throw into the omelette. Generally, I like to prepare as much as I can a week in advance to keep me on track. At about ten-thirty or eleven I'll have the milk serving. If I haven't eaten the fruit earlier sometimes I'll have the fruit then, one of my favorite food combinations. In the winter I know I need hot food, so the menu will be different. And so on throughout the day, I "break up" breakfast, lunch, and dinner and pay special attention to the time of year to make sure the foods will "do it" for me. My main meal is between 2:00 PM and 3:00 PM because that's when my energy level is lowest. I'm not a night eater, so I never have to "leave over" much for the evening.

A woman in my group who loves bread stretches it out by creating all kinds of delicious vegetable sandwiches on rye bread. She knows that a slice or two of bread will not satisfy her, so she uses the vegetables to give her the full feeling she needs. A man in the group does the same thing, only he uses vegetables to stretch out his meat portion.

Pay attention to your food needs, and you'll find that the desire to binge will diminish.

CHAPTER ELEVEN

A Final Recipe for Success

Nobody stays the same.

A woman in my group told me the following story the other day and it made an impression on me because it summed up the way change takes place. "A neighbor brought me a bag of pistachio nuts for the Chinese New Year. I didn't even know it was the Chinese New Year, but I was ready to celebrate it right away! That was my first impulse. 'I love pistachio nuts—I'll finish them off.' But then I thought: *This is the old me.*

"My second impulse was to throw away the bag of nuts as soon as she left. After all, I was doing so well on program. I'd lost three pounds that month. But then I thought: *This is the old me.*

"My third—I won't say "impulse" because it wasn't an impulse but a carefully reasoned solution—was to look up the value of pistachio nuts in the food lists and divide the bag up into seven portions which I would have over the week as a daily treat. And I was really surprised at myself and thought: *This is the new me.*"

Creating that "new me" of hers took time and effort—this woman has been a member for a number of years—but isn't it worth it when you can achieve results like that? Nothing is certain, but you just know that this kind of change has a better chance of being long-lasting.

By nature, I'm a perfectionist. I drive myself and everybody around me crazy sometimes. If I buy a breakfront for my living room, it has to look just right—I waited fifteen years until I found exactly what I was looking for. When I have a dress or a suit tailored, it must look perfect. When my children were sick, who watched over them all night? That is who I am. All or nothing. But when it comes to food, I've had to learn the hard way that that just doesn't work. Just as important as learning not to overindulge, I've had to learn to indulge occasionally and—I was going to say *Forgive myself for it*—but what I should say is—*Not feel guilty about it*. That was my biggest challenge. Others have different challenges, but the principle is the same: if you are tenacious, if you don't give up, you can build on your strengths and overcome your weaknesses.

The stories in this book are of people whose lives are works-in-progress. You don't stop changing as long as you live. But too often people only have eyes for the finished product. They don't appreciate the victories along the way. And so they become discouraged, and give up. They mourn instead of celebrate!

I'd like to leave you with this final story. Recently, I was at the wedding of the daughter of a close friend of mine. The food was delicious and so I'd gone back for second helpings at the smorgasbord. A woman sitting near me who didn't know me said, "Oh, you thin people! You're so lucky! If I just *looked* at what you're eating, I'd gain weight."

"Excuse me?" I said—not because I hadn't heard her, but because I wanted to hear her say it again. How sweet it was!